THE GREAT PHYSICIAN

A Christian Perspective on Healthcare

ALDO RUBAN A

Contents

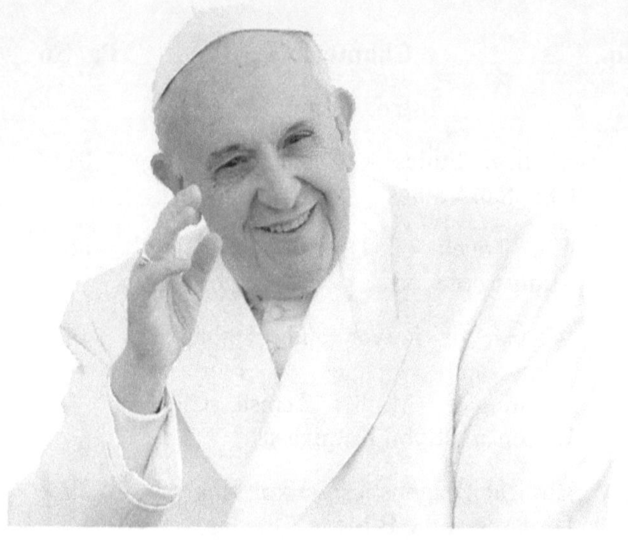

"He is the Good Shepherd, who cares for the wounded sheep and comforts the sick. He is the Good Samaritan who does not pass by the injured person at the roadside, but rather, moved by compassion, cures and attends to him. The Christian medical tradition has always been inspired by the parable of the Good Samaritan"

– Pope Francis

Foreword

Illness and its remedies have been a concern perhaps right from the beginning of human civilization. For instance, the Sumerians are said to have used herbs as medicine almost 5000 years ago. Of course, the field of medicine has become a part of science in our times. Apart from that, it has also been largely commercialized at least since a half century, if not earlier. Hence arises the need for ethics and spirituality in the field of medical science.

The author of this book, Aldo Ruban A, has accomplished a great work in the field of medical spirituality. Meidical spirituality is not alien to medical ethics because there is no spirituality without ethics, and ethics and spirituality go hand in hand together. In fact, ethics is the secular form of spirituality. This book examines illness and its cure from biblical and phenomenological perspectives. It also highlights the spiritual depth of some of the medical remedy providers, including some saints.

I am pleased to appreciate and congratulate the author, Aldo Ruban A, for his insightful contribution. May God, the great healer, shower his abundant blessings on the author and the readers of this valuable book.

July 27, 2024   With love and appreciation,

Most Rev. Dr. Albert Anasthas D.D, S.T.D.
Bishop of Kuzhithurai Diocese.

Foreword

As we navigate the complexities of modern medicine, it's easy to forget the profound impact of Christian values on the very fabric of healthcare. From the early Christian communities, care for the sick and marginalized, to the pioneering work of medical missionaries, Christianity has shaped the way today we approach health, healing, and compassion.

In this timely and thought-provoking book, Aldo Ruban A, a Doctor of Pharmacy student, expertly weaves together the Christian theology, medical ethics, and personal sight, offering a rich tapestry of insights and reflections. With sensitivity and depth, the author explores the intersections of faith and medicine, illuminating the ways in which Christian principles can inform and enrich our understanding of healthcare.

Through these pages, you'll encounter stories of hope and resilience, of courage and grace, and of the transformative power of faith in the face of suffering.

May its words inspire and challenge you, and may its message of hope and compassion resonate deeply in your heart.

July 22, 2024

Dr. Alan James
MBBS., MD (FM), DNB (FM),
Assistant Professor,
Department of Forensic Medicine,
Kanyakumari Govt. Medical College & Hospital,
Asaripallam.

Foreword

With great delight, I appreciate Mr. Aldo Ruban for his earnest effort in writing the book "The Great Physician: A Christian Perspective on Health Care." in this book, the author uncovers how the blend of human effort, God's grace, and medicine provides well – being and alleviates human suffering. His vision is a holistic approach to healing; hence, he urges professionals to provide patient – centered care that comprises kindness, empathy, and altruism, without violating the Christian ethical principles that uphold human dignity.

"Doctor Treats, Jesus Heals" is a phrase that beautifully captures the synergy between medical science and spiritual faith. Jesus represents a source of hope, comfort, and miraculous healing. The author does not portray the healing power of Jesus as a replacement for medical treatment but rather as a complementary force that can enhance the therapeutic relationship and contribute to holistic healing.

It is evident that his book will help readers understand the vital role of medical professionals while also recognizing the spiritual belief in divine intervention and healing.

July 19, 2024   Yours in Christ,

Fr. Dr. S. Xavier Benedict
Vicar General,
Diocese of Kuzhithurai.

Foreword

I am honoured to write this foreword for Aldo Ruban's inspiring book, The Great Physician, which explores the profound truth of Jesus Christ as the Great Physician. As Aldo's Principal and mentor, I have witnessed his growth and passion to share the ethical principles and gospel values for a virtuous living.

This book is a testament to Aldo Ruban's dedication to understanding and conveying the depth of God's love and care for humanity. Through his writing, he skilfully weaves together biblical insights, personal anecdotes, and practical applications, making this book an invaluable resource for anyone seeking spiritual guidance and healing.

Aldo Ruban's unique voice and perspective shines through each page, offering a fresh and compelling exploration of Christ's role as our ultimate Healer. His words will comfort, challenge, and encourage you to deepen your faith and trust in the Great Physician.

I am proud of Aldo Ruban for pursuing his vocation to write this book, and I am confident that it will be a blessing to all who read it. May his words inspire you to experience the transformative power of Jesus Christ in your life.

July 23, 2024

Fr. Dr. John Christopher OIC PhD
Educationalist and Ethicist,
Vice - Provincial Superior,
Bethany Navajeevan Province.

Foreword

I am indeed happy to congratulate Aldo Ruban A, for his wonderful work "The Great Physician", which consists of medical thoughts. It is co-related with the bibilical evidence and its divine elements. Altogether, the book gives us a positive vibration of Jesus, through his words and deeds.

In this era of artificial intelligence, the human world needs more peace and inner joy. Also, more healing is needed for its sustainability. All these thoughts are well developed in this book and it brings out Jesus as a healer and above all, Jesus as a great physician, who is the source of life.

I thank Aldo Ruban for this noble work and wish him many more laurels.

July 19, 2024   Best wishes,

Fr. Dr. Manohiam Xavier
Vicar Forane,
Vencode Vicariate,
Kuzhithurai Diocese.

Foreword

"The Time is always Right

To do what is Right"

> *-   Martin Luther King*

At the right time, with right intension, Mr. Aldo Ruban A, the author of this book emphatically gives his mind to humanity through this book named "The Great Physician".

Jesus, 'The Great Physician', imbibed the principle of medical ethics not as mere words, but He applied it in his day-to-day life for the well being of humanity in all the possible ways.

I, as the Parochial Administrator of St. Francis Xavier's Forane Church at Vencode, wish him all the best for this great effort. Let his vision spread through out this world through this work with the blessings and love of "The Great Physician - CHRIST!"

July 17, 2024

Fr. A. Amal Raj,
Parochial Administrator,
St. Francis Xavier's Forane Church,
Vencode.

Preface

As a Christian and a medical student, I have often grappled with the intersection of my faith and my studies. How can I reconcile the compassionate teachings of Jesus with the scientific rigor of modern medicine? How can I honor God's sovereignty while also taking responsibility for patients' care?

This book is my attempt to explore these questions and uncover the rich connections between Christianity and medicine. Through a combination of biblical reflections, personal anecdotes, and expert insights, I aim to show how our Christian faith can inform and enrich our approach to healthcare.

From the miraculous healings of Jesus to the selfless service of medical missionaries, Christianity has a long history of compassion and care for the sick and suffering. Yet, in today's fast-paced and often secular medical landscape, it can be easy to lose sight of our spiritual roots.

My hope is that this book will inspire and equip Christian healthcare students and professionals to integrate their faith, learning and practice in a way that honors God and benefits the patients. May we be guided by the Great Physician himself, who came to bring healing and wholeness to body, mind, and spirit.

Aldo Ruban A
aldoruban1209@gmail.com

Acknowledgement

Words cannot express my heartfelt gratitude to the following individuals, who played a vital role in bringing this book to life.

I thank God, for his grace, mercy and love which flowed through me and onto the pages of this book. My loving family, who supported me throughout the long hours and late nights of writing, for their unwavering love, patience and understanding during the long writing process.

Most Rev. Dr. Albert Anasthas, Dr. Alan James, Fr. Dr. Xavier Benedict, Fr. Dr. John Christopher, Fr. Dr. Manohiam Xavier and Fr. Amal Raj, for their voice through foreword, are the heart and soul of this book which had made it richer and more meaningful. Mr. Jirilin Babu, my friend, whose guidance and expertise shaped the direction of this book. The staff at Notion Publication, who worked to refine and perfect the manuscript.

Also, I am thankful to countless individuals who shared their insights and expertise with me during the entire process.

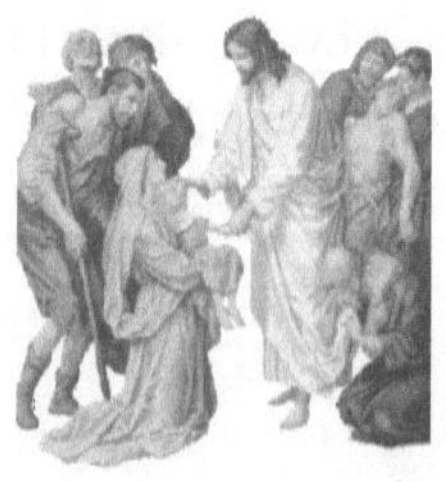

Introduction

Christianity and medicine have been intertwined for centuries, with faith and compassion driving the studies and service of healthcare providers and inspiring countless medical breakthroughs. Yet, in an increasingly secular and complex healthcare landscape, the connection between Christianity and medicine can sometimes seem obscure.

This book seeks to rekindle and deepen that connection, exploring the rich intersections of Christian theology and medical practice. Through a combination of historical reflection, theological analysis, and personal narrative, the book will delve into the ways that Christian principles and values can inform and enrich our understanding of health, healing, and compassion.

From the biblical call to care for the sick and marginalized, to the pioneering work of medical missionaries and faith-based organizations, Christianity has long been a source of inspiration and guidance for healthcare providers, students and patients alike. By examining the ethical and moral dimensions of medical practice and education through the lens of Christian teaching, we can gain a deeper understanding of the human experience and the sacred trust that exists between healthcare providers and those in their care.

Throughout these pages, we will grapple with difficult questions and explore the ways that Christian faith can inform our responses to some of the most pressing challenges in healthcare today.

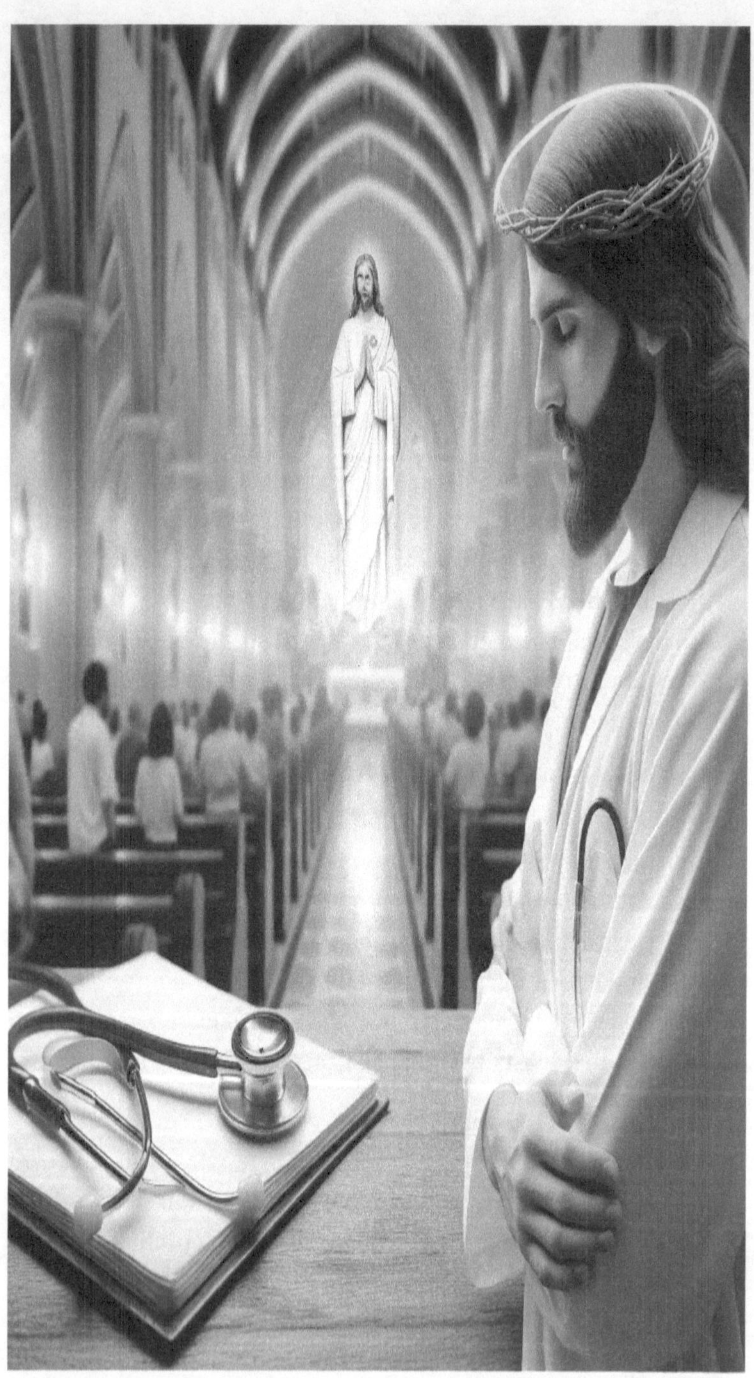

1. Medical Ethics

Correlation with Christian Values

Medical ethics and Christianity share a rich history and common values that guide healthcare professionals in their practice. The four principles of medical ethics – autonomy, beneficence, non-maleficence, and justice – align with Christian teachings and principles.

Autonomy

Autonomy, a fundamental principle in healthcare ethics, respects patients' decision-making capacity and freedom to choose their care. Christianity too, values autonomy, recognizing individuals' God-given free will and moral agency. This content explores the intersection of autonomy and Christianity in healthcare, highlighting their complementary perspectives.

In healthcare, autonomy empowers patients to make informed decisions about their care, aligning with Christian teachings on free will and personal responsibility (Deuteronomy 30:19). Patients' autonomy is rooted in their inherent dignity and worth, created in God's image (Genesis 1:27). This shared understanding of autonomy fosters a collaborative relationship between healthcare providers and patients, respecting patients' values and choices.

Christianity also emphasizes the importance of informed consent, a crucial aspect of autonomy in healthcare. Patients must be fully informed and able to make decisions free from coercion or manipulation, reflecting the biblical principle of honest and transparent communication (Proverbs 10:9).

However, autonomy is not absolute. Christianity teaches that our freedom is bounded by God's moral framework and our responsibility to love our neighbors (Mark 12:31). In healthcare, this means balancing patients' autonomy with beneficence, ensuring that their choices align with their well-being and the greater good.

Non - Maleficence

Non-maleficence mandates that healthcare professionals must not harm. Christianity similarly emphasizes the importance of avoiding harm and promoting well-being, as seen in the biblical teaching "Do no harm, and do good" (Romans 13:10). Let us explore the intersection of non-maleficence and Christianity in healthcare, highlighting their shared commitment to preventing harm and promoting patient well-being.

In healthcare, non-maleficence is reflected in evidence-based practice, where healthcare professionals prioritize treatments that minimize harm and promote healing. This aligns with Christian teachings on loving one's neighbors (Mark 12:31) and doing unto others as you would have them do unto you (Matthew 7:12). By avoiding harm and promoting well-being, healthcare professionals embody Christian values of compassion, empathy, and kindness.

Christianity also emphasizes the importance of self-care and avoiding harm to oneself. The biblical teaching "love your neighbor as yourself" (Mark 12:31) implies a responsibility to care for one's own well-being, recognizing that self-care is essential to caring for others. Healthcare professionals, therefore, have a Christian imperative to prioritize their own well-being, avoiding burnout and compassion fatigue that could lead to harm themselves or their patients.

However, non-maleficence is not limited to individual actions. Christianity teaches that systemic injustices and structural harm are also contrary to God's will (Isaiah 58:6-7). Healthcare professionals must advocate for policies and practices that promote equity, justice, and access to care, recognizing that healthcare is a fundamental human right.

Beneficence

Beneficence promotes acts of kindness, charity, and compassion. Christianity similarly emphasizes the importance of loving one's neighbors and showing kindness to all (Mark 12:31, Luke 10:25-37). The intersection of beneficence and Christianity in healthcare highlights their shared commitment in promoting patient well-being and alleviating suffering.

In healthcare, beneficence is reflected in acts of compassion, empathy, and kindness. Healthcare professionals demonstrate beneficence by providing care that prioritizes patients' well-being, alleviates suffering, and promotes healing. This aligns with Christian teachings on loving one's neighbors and doing well to all (Galatians 6:10). By showing kindness and compassion, healthcare professionals embody Christian values of love, care, and concern for the well-being of others.

Christianity also emphasizes the importance of selfless service and humility in caring for others. Jesus taught his followers to serve others without expectation of reward or recognition (Matthew 20:26-28). Healthcare professionals, likewise, are called to serve patients with humility and compassion, prioritizing their needs above personal interests.

Moreover, beneficence extends beyond individual acts of kindness to systemic efforts to promote healthcare equity and access. Christianity teaches that caring for the vulnerable and advocating for justice are essential to living out one's faith (Isaiah 58:6-7, Matthew 25:31-46). Healthcare professionals must advocate for policies and practices that promote healthcare as a fundamental human right, accessible to all.

Justice

Justice ensures fair distribution of resources and access to care. Christianity similarly emphasizes the importance of justice, compassion, and care for the vulnerable (Isaiah 58:6-7, Matthew 25:31-46). The intersection of justice and Christianity in healthcare highlights their shared commitment to promote equitable access to care and addressing systemic injustices.

In healthcare, justice is reflected in the allocation of resources, prioritizing those most in need. Christianity teaches that all individuals are created equal in God's eyes (Galatians 3:28) and deserve access to care regardless of race, gender, or socioeconomic status. Healthcare professionals must advocate for policies and practices that promote healthcare equity, challenging systemic barriers and discrimination.

Christianity also emphasizes the importance of caring for the marginalized and vulnerable, including the poor, widows, and orphans (James 1:27). Healthcare professionals are called to serve these populations with compassion and advocacy, addressing social determinants of health and promoting health equity.

Moreover, justice in healthcare requires addressing systemic issues like healthcare disparities, unequal access, and discrimination. Christianity teaches that faith without works is dead (James 2:26) and that true religion involves caring for the oppressed and vulnerable (James 1:27). Healthcare professionals must work towards creating a just healthcare system that prioritizes the needs of all individuals, particularly those marginalized.

Ultimately, the intersection of these four pillars of medical ethics and Christianity in healthcare underscores the importance of compassionate, patient-centered care that prioritizes kindness, empathy, and altruism. By embracing this shared commitment, healthcare professionals can provide care that honors the dignity and worth of every individual, reflecting God's love and care for all creation.

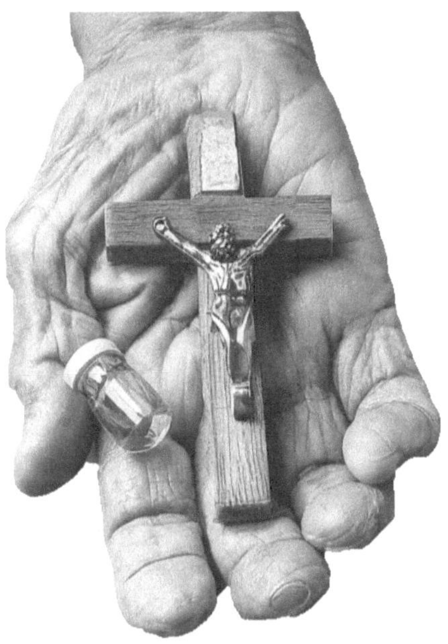

2. The Touch of Divine

Healing Ministry Of God

This chapter sets the stage for exploring the healing ministry of God, emphasizing His compassion, power, and authority over sin and sickness. It also invites readers to reflect on their own brokenness and seek restoration, highlighting the promise of abundant life through Jesus' teachings and sacrifice.

Jesus Christ, the Great Physician, came to heal the whole person - body, mind, and spirit. Throughout His earthly ministry, He demonstrated a profound compassion for those suffering from various afflictions, restoring health and wholeness to countless individuals. From the blind man who received sight to the woman who touched His hem and was freed from her affliction, Jesus' healing touch was a manifestation of God's love and grace.

The healing ministry of Christ is a testament to His power and authority over sin, sickness, and death. It is a reminder that our bodies are temples of the Holy Spirit, worthy of care and respect. As we explore the healing ministry of Christ, we are invited to confront our own brokenness, to seek His restoration, and to embrace His promise of abundant life.

As we delve into the stories of Jesus' healing ministry, may we encounter the loving touch of the Great Physician, and may our faith be strengthened to receive His healing grace in our lives.

Raising of Lazarus from Dead

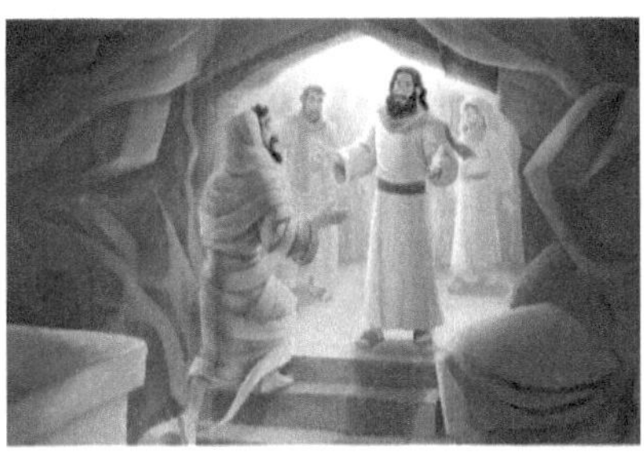

"Did I not tell you that if you believe, you will see the glory of God?" - John (11:40)

The Raising of Lazarus is one of the most remarkable miracles recorded in the Bible, demonstrating Jesus' power over death and his divine authority. According to the Gospel of John (Chapter 11), Lazarus, a close friend of Jesus and brother of Mary and Martha, fell ill and passed away. Despite being informed of Lazarus' critical condition, Jesus delayed his visit to Bethany, arriving four days after Lazarus' burial.

At the moment Jesus arrived Bethany, he noticed that Lazarus became lifeless and had already been inside the tomb for the past 4 days. He first met Martha and Mary. Martha lamented that Jesus did not arrive soon enough to heal her brother ("if you had been here, my brother would not have died") and Jesus replied with the familiar statement, "I am the resurrection, and the life. He who believeth in me, though he were dead, yet shall he live: And whosoever liveth and believeth in me shall never die". Martha actually believed and stated, "Yes, Lord. I believe that you are the Messiah, the Son of God, who has to come into the world". Jesus, moved by their sorrow and faith, proceeded to the tomb, prayed, and commanded Lazarus to come out. To the amazement of the mourners, Lazarus emerged from the tomb, still wrapped in his burial cloths.

This miracle showcased Jesus' divine authority and power over death, foreshadowing his own resurrection and the promise of eternal life for believers. The raising of Lazarus also demonstrated Jesus' compassion and empathy, as he wept alongside Mary and Martha, sharing in their sorrow.

Through this extraordinary event, Jesus revealed his glory and reinforced his message of hope, redemption, and the triumph over death. The Raising of Lazarus remains a powerful symbol of the Christian faith, inspiring generations to trust in Jesus' promises and resurrection power.

The Haemorrhaging Women

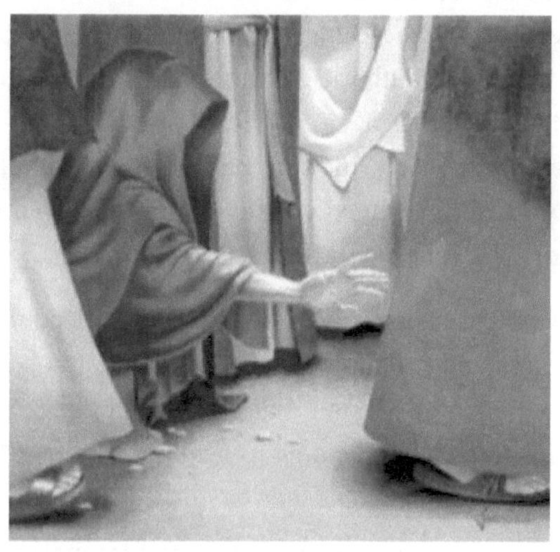

"Daughter, your faith has healed you. Go in peace and be freed from your suffering" - (Mark 5:34)

The story of this woman took place within a larger story. On his journey to a religious leader's house to heal his dying daughter, Jesus met a woman who had bleeding disorder and the issue had continued for the past twelve years. That's a very long time. She had spent all her wealth on treatments from many doctors, and nothing had helped her. In fact, bleeding had grown worse (Mark 5:25–26). The Jewish Law declared her to be ceremonially unclean due to her bleeding issue (Leviticus 15:25-27). This indicates that she would not have been permitted to enter the temple for Jewish religious ceremonies. According to the Decree, anything or any person she touched turned out to be unclean.

The point that she was in the crowd around Jesus means that everyone who bumped into her would have become unclean, together with Jesus. But, after twelve years of suffering, she was obviously despairing for a miracle. "When she heard about Jesus, she came up behind him in the crowd and touched his cloak, because she thought, 'If I just touch his clothes, I will be healed'" (Mark 5:27–28).

As soon as the woman touched Jesus, he responded to the woman who touched His cloak and was healed. People were pushing into Him from all around. Yet, He stopped, turned, and asked, "Who touched my clothes?" (Mark 5:30). The disciples were skeptical, but Jesus knew that healing power had gone out of Him. We can't "steal" a miracle from God. After the woman came forward and explained herself, Jesus cleared her delusions about healing, saying, "Daughter, your faith has healed you. Go in peace and be freed from your suffering" (Mark 5:34). At that very moment, Jesus did what doctors in twelve years had not been able to. This proves the healing power of Christ.

The Paralyzed Man

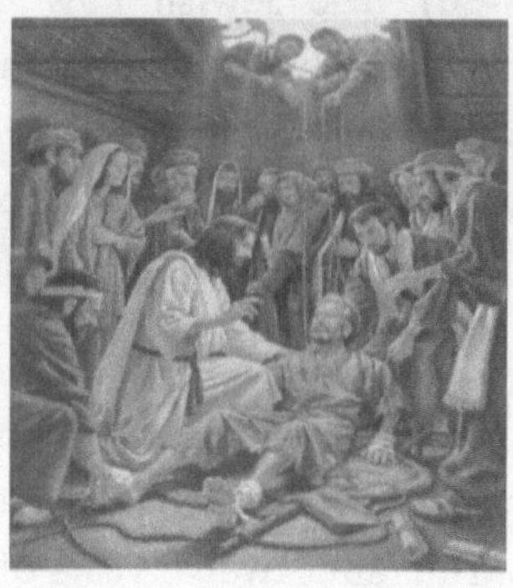

"Get up, take up your bed, and walk." - (John 5:8)

John's Gospel describes Jesus, visiting Jerusalem for a Jewish feast (John 5:1), encountered a man who had been paralyzed for thirty-eight years. Jesus asked the man whether he wants to get well. The man explained that he was unable to enter the water, because he had no one to help him in and others go down ahead of him. Jesus asked him to pick up his bed and walk; the man was promptly cured.

The Gospel reveals that this healing took place on the Sabbath, and the local Jews told the cured man that the Law preclude him to carry his mat on Sabbath. He answered them that he had been instructed to do so by the man who had healed him. They enquired him whom that healer was; but as Jesus had slipped away into the crowd, he was unable to recognize him.

Later, Jesus found the man in the Temple, and told him not to sin again, so that nothing worse would happen to him. The man went away and told the Jewish people that it was Jesus who had made him well (John 5:15). The Gospel explains that the Jews began to persecute Jesus because he was healing on the Sabbath. He responded by quoting that "My Father is still working, and I also am working" (John 5:17). This assertion made the Jews more determined to kill him, because not only is he breaking the Sabbath but he is making himself equal to God by calling God his father (John 5:1–18).

Naaman Healed of Leprosy

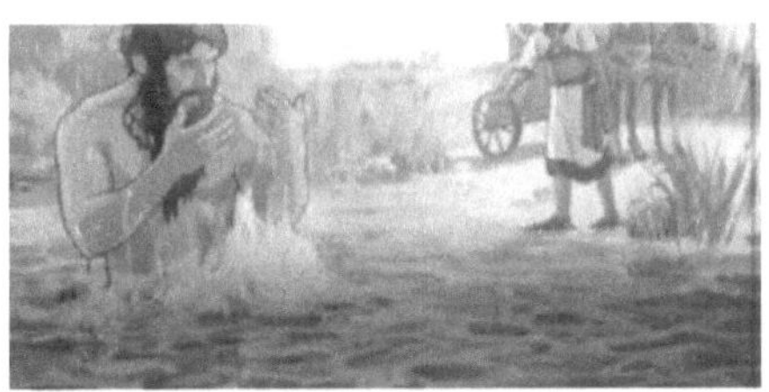

"Go and wash in the Jordan River seven times, and your flesh will be restored to you and you shall be clean."
- (2 Kings 5:10)

Naaman was a brave man and the commander of the army of the king of Syria who was a leper in need of healing as mentioned in the scripture. Having skin lesions as its primary external sign, Leprosy is a granulomatous disease of peripheral nerves and mucosa of the upper respiratory tract.. If left untreated, leprosy may cause permanent damage to the skin, nerves, limbs, and eyes.

Naaman was in need of healing that medical science could not provide. He needed a healing that is possible only through the miracle healing power of God.   In 2 Kings 5:1-19, Naaman was sent to Elisha, a mighty prophet of God to be healed supernaturally. Instead of Elisha coming directly to greet Naaman, he sent a messenger to him saying, "Go and wash in the Jordan River seven times, and your flesh will be restored to you and you shall be clean."

Naaman was livid with the message. Because he expected Elisha to greet him, lay hands on him and miraculously heal leprosy. Naaman finally bowed himself in complete obedience to the loving commands of God's messenger. By doing so, he was touched and healed by God. The scripture utters". Naaman went down and dipped himself in the Jordan seven times, according to the command of the man of God. Then his skin was restored and became like the skin of a small boy, and he was clean" (2 Kings 5:14).

Raising of the Widow's Son of Nain

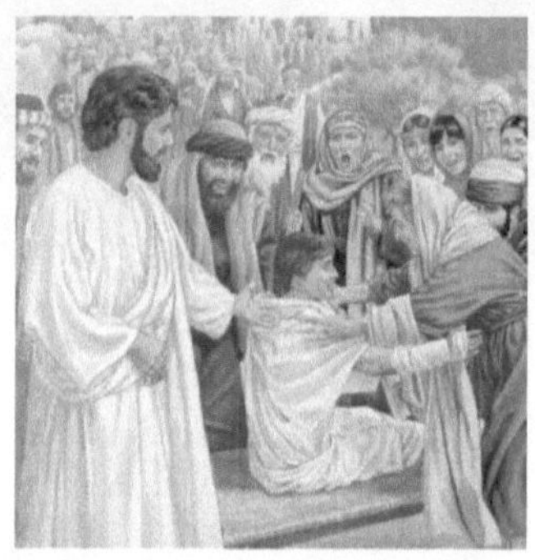

"Young men, I say to you, arise." - (Luke 7:14)

The most reflective of all the miracles Jesus performed during His earthly ministry are those in which He resurrected someone. The New Testament records three of the resurrection miracles, including the raising of widow's son, rising of Jairu's daughter, and of Lazarus. Luke the physician is the only one to recorded the raising of a widow's son (Luke 7:11-17).

One fine day, Jesus and His disciples departed to a town called Nain. Lots of people followed them. As they were walking into the town, they saw a huge group of people carrying a dead man. His mom was crying as he was her only son and she was a widow too.

When Jesus saw her crying, He felt very sad, walked over to her and said, "Don't cry." Then he touched where the dead man was lying on, and everyone stopped moving. Jesus said to the dead man, "Get up!" And the man stood, sat up and started talking. By doing this, Jesus gave back the man to his mom. Everyone was really surprised and scared. They all acclaimed God and said that Jesus was the great prophet sent by God.

Jesus has the power over death and can bring people back to life. Jesus cares about us, for our pains and wants to comfort us. When God does something amazing in our life, it becomes important to praise and give thanks to him.

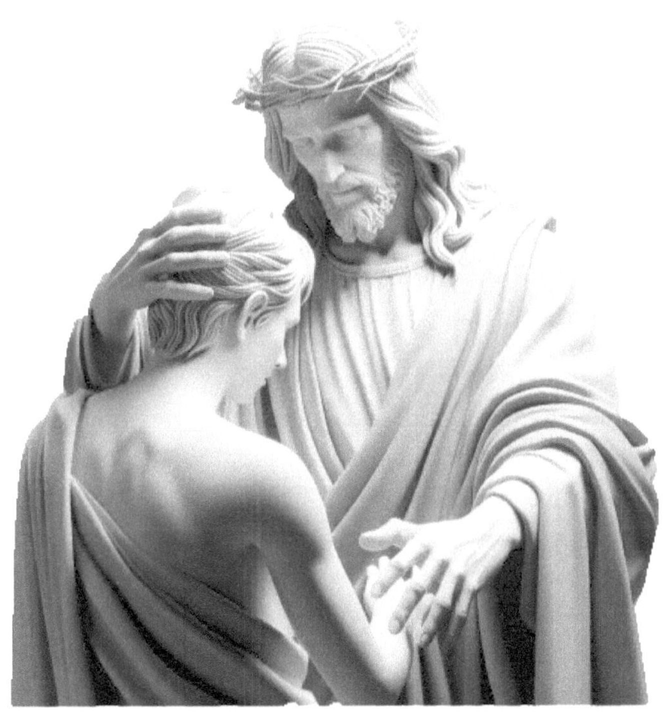

3. Women of Prayer and Healing

Lives and Legacies of Florence Nightingale, Mother Teresa, Clara Barton and Sybil Kathigasu

This chapter sets the stage for exploring the lives and legacies of women who have made significant contributions to healing and spiritual care, highlighting their dedication, compassion, and faith. It invites readers to be inspired by their examples and to continue their work of serving others with love and prayer.

Throughout history, women have played a vital role in the healing and spiritual care of others. From the early Christian martyrs to modern-day healthcare providers, women have been instrumental in bringing comfort, compassion, and hope to all those in need.

This chapter celebrates the lives and legacies of three great women who have dedicated themselves to the powerful combination of healing and prayer. From saints and mystics to nurses and medical missionaries, these women have embodied the tender touch of God's love and the transformative power of prayer.

Florence Nightingale - The Lady with the Lamp

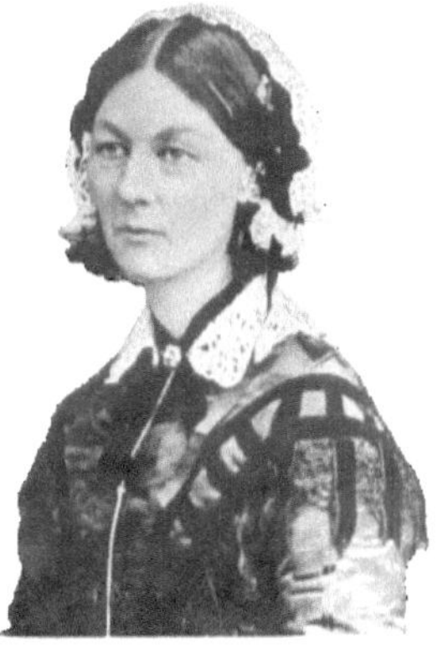

I heard the voice of the Lord saying, "Whom shall I send? And who will go for us?" And I said, "Here am I. Send me!"
- (Isaiah 6:8)

Early Life and Training

Florence Nightingale was born on May 12, 1820, in Florence, Italy and was named after the city of her birth. She was born in an upper-class English family. She was baptized in the Church of England in Florence. Her father William Shore Nightingale was a wealthy landlord and her mother Frances Nightingale, a socialite who hailed from a family of wealthy merchants. From her young age, Florence Nightingale assisted the poor and ill people in her neighboring village, and by the age of 16, she considered nursing to be her life's calling by God.

At her time, nursing was considered a lowly and menial profession in England, and Florence Nightingale's refusal to marry at her 17 years disappointed her parents. In July 1850, Nightingale enrolled herself for training at the Institution of Protestant Deaconesses at Kaiserswerth, Germany. There she discovered basic nursing abilities including the patient observation and good hospital management.

Faith and Biblical Foundations

Nightingale's faith was from her childhood, nourished by wide and regular reading and study of the Bible, the liberal French Dominicans, numerous popular religious novels, biographies of missionaries and saints, tracts from the Society for Promoting Christian Knowledge etc. Nightingale believed that God made the world and runs it by his own laws.

Nightingale acquired significant guidance from the reading of scripture. She believed that God wants us to act and to reflect God's glory to the world through practical achievements.

Nightingale in fact had kept saying, "Here am I, send me", to God for years after her "call to service." Her family did not wanted her to be a nurse. Throughout her life, she greatly appreciated missionaries like David Livingstone for his willingness to go and act for Gods will.

St. Mary's acceptance of her mission, at the annunciation, was her favorite passage, much quoted and widely applied. She considered herself as handmaid of the Lord. May we all answer the angel as Mary did: "Behold the handmaid of the Lord: be it unto me according to Thy word" (Luke 1:38).

Her life of work was nourished by prayer and much devotional reading. She believed that a life of prayer was crucial to support her active healthcare service. She had been described, by a Catholic bishop, as having a Franciscan spirituality.

Recognition and Role in Nursing Education

She was awarded the "Nightingale Jewel," a brooch with an engraved dedication from Queen Victoria, for her service in the Crimean war. She was also granted a prize of 250,000 dollars from the British government and used the money to establish the Nightingale Training School for Nurses and St. Thomas' Hospital. Her work lifted the reputation of nursing from menial to a respectable profession for which many upper-class women desired.

Death

She entered into her eternal life on August 13, 1910, at the age of 90 after living an active, fruitful life in which her concepts and contributions helped to shape the way nursing is practiced today in the western world.

The world has reformed a great deal since Nightingale said to the Lord, "Here am I, send me," and God did!

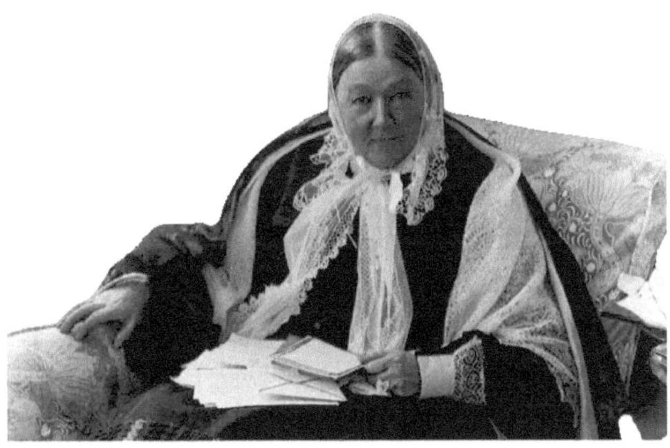

St. Mother Teresa – Angel of Mercy

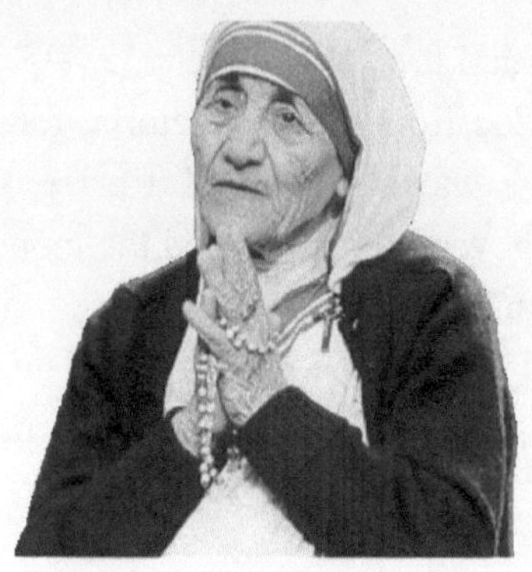

"Truly I tell you, whatever you did for one of the least of these brothers and sisters of mine, you did for me" – Matthew 25:40

Early Life and Vocation

Mother Teresa was born as Agnes Gonxha Bojaxhiu on August 26, 1910, in Skopje, North Macedonia. Her family was of Albanian origin. Her father, a successful merchant, died when she was just eight. After his death, her family struggled economically, but her mother instilled in young Agnes the significance of leading a Christian life and serving the less privileged.

At the age of 12, Agnes first felt the call from god to become a nun and to dedicate her life to Him. She left home at the age of 18 and joined the Sisters of Loreto, an Irish Catholic order which had missions in India. Before traveling to Kolkata, in late 1928, she received training near Dublin, where she began learning English. She took her first vows as a nun in May 1931, and received a new name Teresa, after Saint Theresa of Lisieux. She became known as Mother Teresa from 1937, when she took her final vows.

Healthcare Service

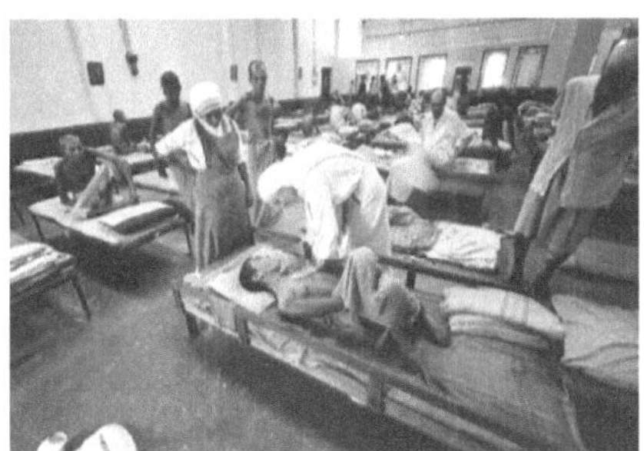

In 1950, Mother Teresa opened a homeopathic dispensary to save the poor in Calcutta. Over time, her "Missionaries of Charity" increased the number of homeopathic dispensaries to four. Mother Teresa was concerned so much on helping the poor that she studied Homeopathy on her own with Dr. Jai Chand, an Indian Homeopathic Physician. She trusted the Sisters and she didn't consider herself as a homeopathic practitioner and left the treatment of patients with chronic illnesses to homeopathic doctors. She educated herself to prescribe for acute illnesses. The Sisters of Charity were there to serve and homeopathy helped them to do treatment inexpensively, effectively, and with pure hearts.

Gandhi said, "Homeopathy cures a greater percentage of medical cases than any other method of treatment. Homeopathy is the latest and refined method of treating patients economically and non-violently."

Mother Teresa, the Saint Who Fought Against Stigma of Leprosy

Mother Teresa established a Leprosy Fund to educate people regarding the disease and established a number of mobile leper clinics in September 1957 to provide affected people with medical aids.

By the mid of 1960s, she instituted a leper colony called Shanti Nagar (The Place of Peace), a place established for lepers to work and live a satisfactory life. Inspired by her meticulous work in creating awareness of the disease, the government offered the land on which the leper colony was built. When Mother Teresa was focusing Kolkata alone, there were about 30,000 lepers, which account half of what the entire nation has today.

In order to expand her service to leprosy patients, she pleads support from the West and private donors. By 1960s, she went on tours to the US and Europe to create awareness about the work her team was doing. The West opened their funds charitably. During 1980s, when the World Health Organization began proposing multi-drug treatment for leprosy, Mother Teresa launched an awareness campaign to educate patients and medical professionals regardingly.

It was possible for her to bring leprosy patients into ordinary, at a time when they were scared, stigmatized and often abandoned by their families. While her motto was to "To do small things with great love", her "small things" left a great influence on the lives of the deprived and needy.

Spiritual Life

In his first encyclical *Deus caritas est* , Pope Benedict XVI mentioned Mother Teresa three times and used her life to clarify one of the main points of the encyclical, "In the example of Blessed Teresa of Calcutta, we have a clear illustration of the fact that time devoted to God in prayer strengthens our loving service to neighbors."

Although her order was not connected with the Franciscan orders, Mother Teresa admired St Francis of Assisi and was influenced by Franciscan spirituality. The Sisters of Charity narrate the prayer of Saint Francis every morning during the thanksgiving after Communion at the Mass. St Francis emphasized scarcity, charity, obedience and surrender to Christ. He devoted much of his life in serving the poor, particularly lepers.

Recognitions and Death

In 1979, she received the Nobel Peace Prize for her humanitarian work, and the following year the Indian government conferred on her the Bharat Ratna, the country's highest civilian honor.

Mother Teresa had a heart attack in Rome (Vatican) in 1983 while she was visiting Pope John Paul II. Subsequent to the second attack in 1989, she was fixed with a pacemaker. she had additional heart problems, after a phase of pneumonia in Mexico in 1991. Although Mother Teresa wished to resign as the superior of the Missionaries of Charity, sisters of the congregation voted for her to remain, and she agreed to continue.

In April 1996, Mother Teresa collapsed, breaking her collarbone, and four months later she had malaria and heart failure again. Though she underwent heart surgery, her health declined. According to the Archbishop of Calcutta Henry Sebastian D'Souza, he ordered a priest to perform an exorcism (with her permission) when she was first hospitalized with cardiac problems because he thought she might be under attack by the devil. On 13 March 1997, Mother Teresa resigned as provincial of the Missionaries of Charity. She entered God's eternal kingdom on 5 September.

At the time of her death in September 1997, Mother Teresa's Missionaries of Charity had over 4,000 sisters operating in 610 missions in 123 countries globally. These included hospitals and homes for people with HIV/AIDS, leprosy and tuberculosis. The Missionaries of Charity was also assisted by co-workers whose count crossed 1 million by the 1990s.

Analyzing her endeavors and achievements, Pope John Paul II said, "From Where did Mother Teresa find the strength and perseverance to dedicate her completely in serving others? She found it in prayer and meditation in Jesus Christ, his Holy Face, his Sacred Heart, and the Holy Eucharist."

In personal, Mother Teresa experienced doubts and struggle in her religious dogmas which lasted nearly 50 years, until the end of her life. Mother Teresa expressed vital doubts about God's existence and pain over her lack of belief. "Where is my faith? Even deep down... there is nothing but emptiness and darkness.... If there be God – please forgive me. When I try to raise my feelings to Heaven, there is such convicting bareness that those feelings return back like sharp knives and hurt my soul".

After ten years of doubt, Mother Teresa described a brief period of renewed faith. After Pope Pius XII's death in 1958, she was praying for him at a requiem mass where she was relieved of "the long darkness… that strange suffering."

Mother Teresa wrote many letters to her confessors and superiors over a 66-year period, most notably to Archbishop of Calcutta Ferdinand Perier and Jesuit priest Celeste van Exem (her spiritual mentor since the formation of the Missionaries of Charity). She wished that her letters be destroyed, worried that "people will think more of me – less of Jesus".

Sainthood

Pope Francis canonized her at a solemn ceremony on 4 September 2016 in St. Peter's Square in the Vatican City. Tens of thousands of people witnessed the ceremony, including 15 government delegations and 1,500 homeless people from all across Italy.

After the canonization, Mother Teresa is known as St. Teresa of Calcutta. Her feast day is celebrated on September 5. She is the patron saint of World Youth Day, the Missionaries of Charity, and co-patron of the Archdiocese of Calcutta.

Clara Barton - Angel of the Battlefield

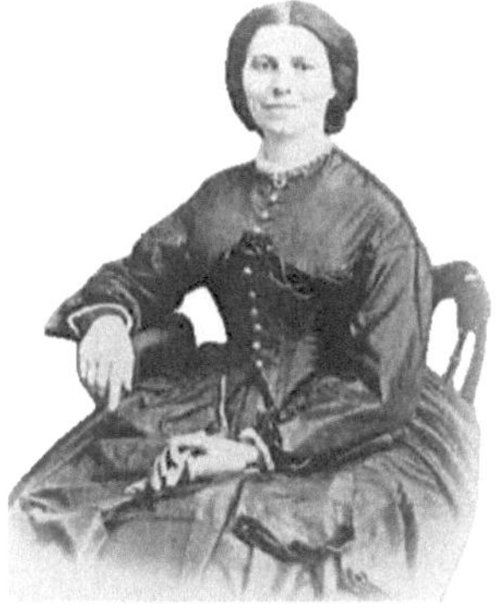

"We are God's handiwork, created in Christ Jesus to do good works" - Ephesians 2:10

Early Life

Clarissa Harlowe Barton was born on Christmas day, 1821, in North Oxford, Massachusetts. Clara Barton was the fifth child of Stephen and Sarah Barton. Her first experience with nursing was as a girl when she tended her older brother who had a head injury. After an early career in teaching, where she founded a free public school in New Jersey, Clara moved to Washington, D.C., and worked at the U.S. Patent Office. She was one of the first women to work for the federal government.

Service at the Battlefield

Clara was still living in Washington when the American Civil War began in 1861. During that time, she bravely provided nursing care and supplies to soldiers — activities that ultimately defined her life and earned her the nickname, Angel of the Battlefield. She traveled with the Union Army bringing surgical supplies, cooking, and tending the wounded. The tale is told of Barton holding an injured soldier when a bullet ripped through her sleeve and into the man, killing him. She later pondered, "I have never mended that hole in my sleeve. I wonder if a soldier ever does mend a bullet hole in his coat." One essential service Clara performed was to record personal information of the soldiers. She wrote to family members of missing, wounded, and dead soldiers. When the war ended, Clara found new ways to help the military. With permission from President Lincoln, she opened the Office of Missing Soldiers, helping to reconnect more than 20,000 soldiers with their families.

Barton then traveled to Switzerland for rest, where she learned about the Red Cross movement, a European humanitarian effort to provide neutral aid to those injured in combat. Inspired by that cause, Clara volunteered with the International Committee of the Red Cross, providing civilian relief during the Franco-Prussian War. This experience, along with her work during the Civil War, inspired Clara to bring the Red Cross movement to America.

Founding the American Red Cross

On May 21, 1881, Clara founded the American Red Cross, and by 1882, the U.S. ratified the Geneva Conventions — laws that, to this day, protect the war-wounded and civilians in conflict zones. This later resulted in a U.S. congressional charter, officially recognizing Red Cross services.

Spiritual Life

Early on, Barton realized, "we are God's handiwork, created in Christ Jesus to do good works, which God prepared in advance for us to do." (Ephesians 2:10) She followed the path God set before her, amidst danger and opposition. She supported equal rights and was willing to help anyone regardless of race, gender, or station. She lived out the Galatians 3:28 reminder, "There is neither Jew nor Gentile, neither slave nor free, nor is there male and female, for you are all one in Christ Jesus." Her tireless work brought aid and comfort to men on the battlefield, to families in disasters, and helped provide supplies for first responders during her life and beyond.

She persevered, trusting that "God, who began the good work within you, will continue his work until it is finally finished..." (Philippians 1:6)

Death

Clara Barton served as Red Cross president for 23 years, retiring in 1904. After a lifetime of service, Clara died at her home in Glen Echo, Maryland, on April 12, 1912.

Sybil Kathigasu- Faith amid Torture

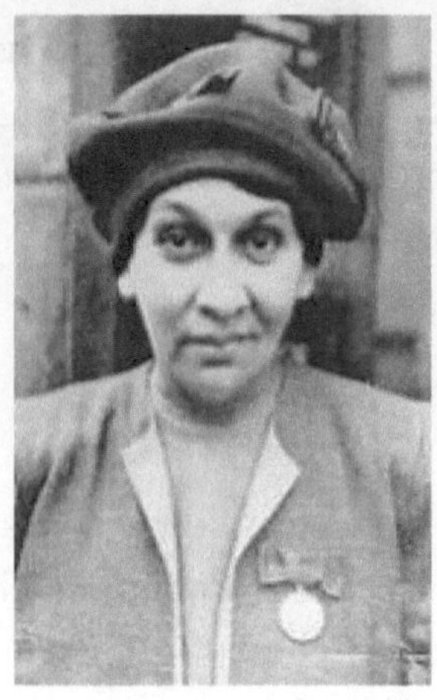

*"The poor and sick are the heart of God. In serving them, we
serve Jesus Christ" - St. Camillus de Lellis*

Sybil Medan Kathigasu neè Daly, a nurse and resistance fighter
during the Second World War, is little known even within
Malaysia, the country she helped during its occupation by
Japanese forces. But in my opinion her contributions, and her
bravery in the face of hardship, should not be taken lightly or be
forgotten.

Early Life (1899-1920)

Sybil Kathigasu was born on September 7, 1899, in Medan,
Sumatra, Dutch East Indies (now Indonesia), to a Eurasian
family of Portuguese and Malay descent. Her father, Allan
Kathigasu, was a British colonial officer, and her mother, Maria
Gonzales, was a nurse.

Sybil grew up in a close-knit family with two younger
siblings. She received her early education at the Convent School

in Medan, where she excelled in academics and developed a strong interest in medicine.

Nursing Career (1920-1942)

In 1920, Sybil moved to Singapore to pursue a career in nursing at the General Hospital. She trained under the British colonial medical system and became a skilled nurse and midwife.

While embarking on her nursing and midwifery course at the General Hospital in Kuala Lumpur, she encountered and fell in love with one of the doctors there, a Dr. Arumugam Kanapathi Pillay. He was said to be a quiet reserved man, which was in contrast to Sybil's more outgoing nature. Despite being in love there was initial objection from Sybil's family due to Sybil's family being Catholic while he was a Hindu. Eventually, he converted and changed his name to Abdon Clement Kathigasu, three days before they finally wedded on January 7th 1919 in St. John's Church in Kuala Lumpur. By the time they started their own practice in Ipoh in April 1921, Sybil had given birth to two children Michael and Olga, though Michael died due to complications not long after birth, and adopted another child named William. Another child, Dawn, was born in 1936.

They worked together in various hospitals in Malaya, providing medical care to the local population.

World War II and Resistance (1942-1945)

During World War II, Sybil and her family remained in Malaya, where they witnessed the Japanese occupation. Despite the risks, Sybil continued to provide medical care to those in need, including resistance fighters.

In 1943, Sybil joined the Malayan People's Anti-Japanese Army (MPAJA), a resistance movement fighting against the Japanese occupation. She provided medical support to the resistance fighters and helped establish a network of underground hospitals both Sybil and her husband were arrested in August 1943. They were imprisoned in Bath Gajah jail where they were tortured for any information they had on the rebel troops. Despite the ghastly torture, Sybil refused to say anything to her captors. This continued until February 1945 where they were sentenced in a kangaroo court trial for a variety of crimes including working with the rebels, leading to a 15 year sentence for her husband and a life sentence for Sybil herself.

The couple were found and freed from their imprisonment in August 1945 soon after Malaya was liberated from the occupation, and not long after that was Sybil flown to the United Kingdom so that her injuries could be treated. While there she went about writing a memoir of her experiences of the war, later collected and published in 1954 under the name No Dram of Mercy. She was also awarded the George Medal for Gallantry by King George VI, the only Malayan woman to have received the honour. Unfortunately her injuries were too severe and she died in Scotland on June 12th 1948. She was initially buried there before having her remains brought back to Ipoh and reburied in St. Michael's Church Cemetery on March 21, 1949 with the honour of a grand funeral procession.

Process of Beatification

In a diocesan notification issued on July 1, Cardinal Sebastian Francis, Bishop of Penang, noted that Kathigasu's life continues to inspire people even 76 years after her death. The Diocese of Penang in Malaysia has officially opened the cause of beatification and canonization for Sybil Kathigasu.

4. Biblical Diagnostics

Exploring the Diseases of the Bible

The sacred text revered by millions, contains numerous accounts of diseases and afflictions that plagued humanity in ancient times. These diseases, often described in vivid detail, were not only physical ailments but also spiritual and emotional afflictions that resonated with the people of that era. The text contains stories, teachings, and wisdom that have guided humanity for centuries. While it is not a medical textbook, it does contain descriptions of various physical ailments and afflictions that were prevalent in ancient times.

In the Bible, diseases were often seen as punishments from God, consequences of sin, or tests of faith. However, they also served as opportunities for healing, redemption, and spiritual growth. From the plagues of Egypt to the healing miracles of Jesus, diseases play a significant role in the biblical narrative.

This introduction sets the stage for an exploration of "Biblical Diagnostics", a journey delves into the historical, cultural, and spiritual contexts of various afflictions mentioned in the Scriptures. Here, we will examine the biblical accounts, their interpretations, and the insights they offer into human nature, suffering, and the divine.

Join me on this fascinating journey as we uncover the stories, meanings, and significance of diseases in the Bible, shedding light on the human experience and the timeless wisdom of Scripture.

Alcoholism- Battling the Bottle

Alcoholism is a chronic and debilitating disease that affects millions of people worldwide. While the term "alcoholism" is not explicitly mentioned in the Bible, the Scriptures contain numerous accounts of excessive drinking and its consequences, which align with the modern understanding of alcoholism as a disease. This essay will explore the biblical perspective on alcoholism, examining the historical and cultural context of drinking in ancient Israel, the physical and spiritual consequences of excessive drinking, and the biblical emphasis on moderation and self-control.

The Bible describes the physical consequences of excessive drinking, including impaired judgment (Genesis 9:21), poor health (Proverbs 23:29-35), and even death (Isaiah 5:11). These consequences align with the modern understanding of alcoholism as a disease that affects physical health. Excessive drinking is also portrayed as a spiritual problem, leading to spiritual decay and separation from God (Isaiah 5:11, 22-23). The Bible emphasizes the importance of self-control and moderation in drinking, encouraging believers to avoid excessive behavior that can lead to harm. The Bible emphasizes moderation and self-control in drinking, encouraging believers to avoid excessive behavior that can lead to harm. This emphasis is seen in passages such as Proverbs 20:1 and Ephesians 5:18, which caution against excessive drinking and encourage responsible behavior.

Wine was a very common drink in Biblical days, much as coffee is now. This was good in a country like Israel. Wine was a safe drink because of its alcoholic content. The Bible speaks favorably of wine in several places. When Isaac gave Jacob his blessing (Gen 27:28), he said "May God give you plenty of grain and wine." Then, of course, we have the classical record of Jesus miraculously changing a huge volume of water into wine.

Some scholars seek to show that the wine was really only grape juice. This is improbable, since grape juice would quickly spoil with temperature and living conditions as they were in Biblical days. Wine was definitely wine as we know it today, and it was a good thing for the people of that day. However, it is also true that some Hebrews used wine to excess and got themselves and others in trouble. The Bible repeatedly speaks favorably of wine, but warns frequently and emphatically against its excessive use.

There seems to be a strange chemistry in the bodies of certain people that produces a strong craving for alcohol. They start drinking it in normal manner with their food, or socially, but are unable to control themselves and go on to excess. Beer and whiskey were probably unknown to the Jews, but excessive wine drinking can do just as much damage as other forms of alcohol intake. Alcohol is a sad looking specimen of humanity, and is on his way to committing suicide through destruction of his brain, liver and other organs.

In modern times alcoholism is looked upon as a disease, and is treated as such. In Biblical days it was considered a moral problem. Chronic alcoholism is an amazingly stubborn ailment. Persons who seem to have recovered from it show relapses after months or years in seventy-five percent of such cases. Christian faith is of enormous help. Several chronic alcoholics have been instantaneously cured of alcoholism by simply accepting Jesus as their Savior and Lord. Undoubtedly there were cases like that in the old days when alcoholics returned to sincere Jehovah worship. Medication, counseling, institutional training, and Alcoholics Anonymous are valuable, but none are as effective as that mysterious experience known as "rebirth."

Blindness

Blindness is a condition characterized by the loss of vision, either partial or total. The Bible describes blindness as a physical affliction in several instances. For example, in Exodus 4:11, God strikes Moses' sister Miriam with leprosy, which results in blindness. Similarly, in 2 Kings 6:18-20, the Aramean army is struck with blindness by God.

Blindness is also used as a symbol of spiritual decay or rebellion in the Bible. For example, in Isaiah 6:9-10, God declares, "Be ever hearing, but never understanding; be ever seeing, but never perceiving." This passage describes spiritual blindness as a result of rebellion against God. Similarly, in Matthew 23:16-26, Jesus condemns the Pharisees for their spiritual blindness, declaring, "You are blind guides leading the blind." Blindness is also described as a manifestation of God's judgment in the Bible. For example, in Leviticus 26:18-19, God declares, "If you do not obey me, I will bring darkness upon you, and your eyes will be so blind that you will grope about like the blind." Similarly, in Revelation 3:17-18, Jesus declares, "You say, 'I am rich; I have acquired wealth and do not need a thing.' But you do not realize that you are wretched, pitiful, poor, blind and naked."

Blindness was common in Egypt, Israel and the Arabian countries. Poverty, unsanitary conditions, brilliant sunlight, excessive heat, blowing sand, accidents, and war injuries were some of the factors involved, but the main cause was ignorance of infectious organisms.

The blindness from birth, spoken of in the Bible was probably ophthalmia neonatorum (gonorrhea of the eyes). This has been the prime cause of infantile blindness for centuries. Women often harbor gonorrheal diplococci in their vaginas, even though they may be totally unaware of the infection. Then, when a baby is born, and it makes its passage down from the uterus, it may get some of the germs in its eyes. The conjunctiva of a baby is an ideal breeding place for gonococci, and in about three days the baby's eyes run with pus. In many cases, permanent blindness results. In modern practice, antiseptic drops are placed in the infant's eyes immediately after birth, and the infective organisms that may be present are destroyed.

The other frequent cause of blindness is trachoma. The infecting organism is a virus. Indians with this disease come in with their bleary, itching, painful eyes. Some of them had an apron of tissue, called a pannus, growing down over the cornea. Many older people had badly deformed eyelids, and some were blind. Today's sulfa drugs provide an easy and complete cure, but in former days it was a devastating illness. In modern medicine, blindness is typically considered a symptom of various underlying medical conditions, such as cataracts, glaucoma, or macular degeneration. Blindness can also be caused by injuries, infections, or genetic disorders.

Boils

It is likely that the word "boil" as used in the Bible covered many types of skin diseases, such as pustules, simple boils, carbuncles, abscesses and infected glands. The Bible describes boils as a physical affliction in several instances. For example, in Exodus 9:9-11, the Egyptians are struck with boils as part of the ten plagues. Similarly, in Job 2:7-8, Job is afflicted with painful boils from head to foot.

Boils are also used as a symbol of spiritual decay or rebellion in the Bible. For example, in Leviticus 13:18-23, the priestly code describes boils as a symptom of spiritual uncleanness. Similarly, in 2 Samuel 3:29, Joab's murder of Abner is punished with a boil that will not heal. In 1 Samuel 5:6-12, the Philistines are struck with boils as punishment for capturing the Ark of the Covenant. Similarly, in Isaiah 1:5-6, God declares, "Why should you be beaten anymore, you rebellious children? Why do you persist in rebellion? Your head is injured, your heart is sick. From head to foot, there is no soundness—only wounds and welts and festering sores."

Boils, as we know them today, are usually caused by staphylococci. These germs are normally present on the surface of the skin, and do no harm unless there is some kind of injury to the skin, allowing the germs to get inside and proliferate. The body reacts with its defense of leucocytes, and in the battle that ensues germs, leucocytes and debris may form a painful pocket of pus that we call a boil. If the boil is single and comes to a head, it ruptures and recovery follows.

A carbuncle is much like a collection of boils in a limited area. The infection runs deeper than an ordinary boil and has several openings. It is commonly located in the back of the neck. It usually covers an area several inches in diameter, and sometimes is fatal.

An abscess may be minor, but frequently is deep, involving important structures of the body, such as muscles, lungs, brain, liver, spleen, kidney, bowel and appendix. Hezekiah's boil must have been a carbuncle or deep abscess, as his life hung in the balance when he was afflicted with it. Job's boils were superficial, or they would have resulted in his death. The boils of the sixth Egyptian plague probably were extremely painful superficial boils.

The Babylonians used boils in its broader sense. Recently archeologists dug up a Babylonian tablet which stated that if a physician cut into a boil and the patient died, the physician would have both his hands cut off. If the patient happened to be a slave, the physician's hands were spared, but he had to buy another slave for the owner of the patient. So, the doctor had to be extremely careful when he lanced an abscess or a boil. In modern medicine, boils are typically considered a symptom of various underlying medical conditions, such as abscesses, cellulitis, or MRSA infections. Boils can also be caused by ingrown hairs, clogged pores, or bacterial infections.

Deafness

Deafness is a topic that is addressed in the Bible, although it is not a prominent theme. However, there are several instances where deafness is mentioned, often in the context of healing miracles performed by Jesus or other biblical figures.

In the Old Testament, deafness is often associated with spiritual deafness, symbolizing a lack of understanding or refusal to listen to God's word. For example, in Isaiah 6:9-10, the prophet Isaiah is instructed by God to speak to the people, but to also tell them that they will not understand or hear, emphasizing their spiritual deafness.

In the New Testament, Jesus heals several individuals who are deaf or have hearing impairments. For instance, in Mark 7:31-37, Jesus heals a deaf man by putting his fingers in the man's ears and saying "Ephphatha!" which means "Be opened!" This miracle is significant not only because it shows Jesus' power to heal physical deafness but also because it symbolizes the opening of spiritual ears to hear God's message.

The Bible also mentions deafness in relation to the importance of communication and understanding. In James 1:19, it is written, "My dear brothers and sisters, take note of this: Everyone should be quick to listen, slow to speak, and slow to anger." This verse highlights the value of listening and understanding, even for those who may not be able to hear in the classical sense. Furthermore, the Bible teaches compassion and inclusivity towards individuals with deafness and other disabilities. In Leviticus 19:14, it is written, "Do not curse the deaf or put a stumbling block in front of the blind, but fear your God, and I will be your God." This verse emphasizes the importance of treating all individuals with respect and dignity, regardless of their abilities.

There are several general areas that may be involved in deafness. The first of these is the external ear canal. With the sand, dust and drying heat of the mid-East, there must have been many cases in which the ear canal became plugged with wax and dirt, producing a serious degree of deafness. Undoubtedly many persons suffered deafness much of their lives because of dirty ears. Infections of the external ear canal were also common in tropical and semi-tropical countries.

The middle ear is another frequent source of trouble. This little chamber with its three tiny ossicles—the malleus, incus and stapes—forming a little chain from the ear drum to the window of the cochlea, and the Eustachian tube coming into it from the pharynx, serves an important function in hearing. The area may become infected by organisms coming through a ruptured ear drum, or through the Eustachian tube. Severe deafness may also be due to the ossicles becoming rigidly solidified to each other following an infection.

The inner ear is the third possible location of trouble. It is called the cochlea because it resembles a snail shell. It is really an extension of the auditory nerve. Infection of the cochlea or tumors of the auditory nerve and hearing center of the brain are uncommon, but severe when they occur. It should be remembered that we have two ears and that it is possible to be deaf in one and not the other.

Dysentery

Dysentery is a bacterial infection that affects the intestines and is characterized by diarrhea, abdominal pain, and blood in the stool. While the Bible does not specifically mention dysentery, it does contain accounts of diseases and afflictions that may be related to dysentery.

In the Old Testament, the Bible describes several instances of plagues and diseases that affected the Israelites, including the plague of hail (Exodus 9:13-35), the plague of locusts (Exodus 10:1-20), and the plague of boils (Exodus 9:9-12). While these plagues are not specifically identified as dysentery, they may have included symptoms similar to those of dysentery.

In the New Testament, Jesus heals several individuals with diseases and afflictions, including a woman with a bleeding disorder (Matthew 9:20-22) and a man with a skin disease (Luke 5:12-14). While these diseases are not specifically identified as dysentery, they may have included symptoms similar to those of dysentery.

The Bible also contains accounts of the Israelites' poor sanitation and hygiene practices, which may have contributed to the spread of diseases like dysentery. For example, in Deuteronomy 23:12-14, the Israelites are commanded to dig a latrine outside the camp and to cover their waste with dirt, to prevent the spread of disease. In addition, the Bible teaches valuable lessons about spiritual cleansing and purification, which may be related to physical cleansing and hygiene. For example, in Leviticus 15:1-33, the Israelites are commanded to wash their bodies and clothes to cleanse themselves from various bodily discharges, including those that may be related to dysentery.

Dysentery was a very common ailment among the people of the mid-East. It was due primarily to three types of organisms—amebae, bacteria and worms. In some cases the body adjusted itself to the invading organism, and there would be only sporadic attacks of diarrhea. But often it was very severe, and at times so bad it was called malignant dysentery. Plague is the most striking example of such malignancy. The stools consisted mainly of mucus, pus and blood. It was accompanied by severe abdominal pain, and frequently high fever. Passage of stools was painful with dysentery because of the irritating effect of the excretions. Hemorrhoids developed, and at times there was a prolapse of the lower part of the colon, as was the case with Jehoram (2 Chron 21:18) "His bowels came out because of the disease, and he died in great agony" (v. 19). There was also rapid loss of weight, and death might ensue within a few days. (Acts 28:8) "Lay sick with fever and dysentery," and we can readily appreciate his gratitude when God healed him.

Fever

Fever is a common symptom of various illnesses and infections, characterized by an elevated body temperature. While the Bible does not specifically mention fever as a distinct medical condition, it contains accounts of individuals with fever-like symptoms and diseases that may be related to fever. Fever refers to bodily temperature distinctly higher than normal. Our bodily temperatures are beautifully controlled under normal circumstances by an inner mechanism which keeps the temperature at about 98.6 degrees Fahrenheit. The controller of this mechanism is a small gland called the hypothalamus, located near the center of the brain. It sends its commands to the liver, heart, lungs, muscles, fat, skin, sweat glands, and other organs, and has them work in unison to keep the body temperature within approximately one degree of the normal 98.6. This temperature control system is another evidence of the supreme intelligence, wisdom and power of God in creation.

Disease may overwhelm this mechanism. When an infecting organism enters the body, a tremendous battle goes on, involving millions of cells, with the body trying desperately to defeat the invading organism. This increases the metabolism of the body and fever results. Usually the body wins and the temperature returns to normal. With extremely severe sickness, the temperature may rise to as high as 108 degrees, and death may ensue.

In the Old Testament, the Bible describes several instances of individuals with high temperatures, sweating, and bodily heat, such as King David (1 Samuel 30:12) and Job (Job 30:27). While these episodes are not specifically identified as fever, they may be related to feverish symptoms. In the New Testament, Jesus heals several individuals with diseases and afflictions, including Peter's mother-in-law who had a "great fever" (Luke 4:38-39). This account is one of the few instances where the Bible specifically mentions fever as a symptom of illness.

The Bible also contains teachings about spiritual purification and cleansing, which may be related to physical health and wellness, including the management of fever. For example, in Matthew 8:14-15, Jesus heals Peter's mother-in-law by touching her hand, highlighting the spiritual dimension of healing and wellness. In addition, the Bible teaches valuable lessons about compassion, understanding, and care for the sick, which are essential for supporting individuals with fever and other illnesses. For example, in Matthew 25:36, Jesus teaches that visiting the sick and caring for their needs is a fundamental aspect of loving one's neighbor as oneself.

Obesity

Obesity is a condition characterized by excess body fat, which can lead to various health problems. While the Bible does not specifically mention obesity as a modern medical diagnosis, it contains accounts of individuals with physical characteristics and behaviors that may be related to obesity.

In the Old Testament, the Bible describes several instances of individuals with large physical stature or excess weight, such as King Saul (1 Samuel 9:2) and Eglon, the king of Moab (Judges 3:17). While these descriptions are not specifically related to obesity, they highlight the physical characteristics of individuals in biblical times.

The Bible also contains teachings about temperance, self-control, and stewardship of the body, which may be related to healthy eating and exercise habits. For example, in 1 Corinthians 6:19-20, Paul writes, "Do you not know that your bodies are temples of the Holy Spirit, who is in you, whom you have received from God? You are not your own; you were bought at a price. Therefore, honor God with your bodies."

Surgeons who have had to cut through two to four inches of fat to get into an abdomen can easily understand what happened to Eglon. Moreover, excessive fat is located not only in a thick, greasy layer between the skin and muscles, but also in the abdomen with its thick mesentery and abundance of fat around the organs.

A panel of doctors from the American Medical Association, testifying in a U.S. Senate Committee hearing, stated that the principal causes of obesity were: 1) heredity, 2) glandular disturbance, 3) nervous worry, and 4) big appetite. Another is the desire for prestige. In countries where food was scarce and an adequate diet difficult to obtain, it was a source of pride to a person if he and the members of his family had full faces and protuberant abdomens. Fatness could be important in a country where the ability to obtain adequate food was uncertain, and the person might have to call on his reserves of fat, much as a camel uses the fat in his hump. In modern times we have been alerted to the dangers of obesity with respect to our hearts, varicose veins, arteriosclerosis, arthritis, diabetes, possible surgery, and the number of years we shall live. Diet and reasonable exercise are the ingredients of relief.

Palsy

Palsy is a general term for paralysis or weakness of the muscles, often accompanied by loss of sensation or control. While the Bible does not specifically mention palsy as a modern medical diagnosis, it contains accounts of individuals with symptoms and conditions that may be related to palsy.

In the New Testament, Jesus heals several individuals with paralysis or weakness, such as the man with the withered hand (Matthew 12:10-13), the paralyzed man lowered through the roof (Mark 2:1-12), and the woman with a spirit of infirmity (Luke 13:10-17). While these accounts are not specifically identified as palsy, they demonstrate Jesus' power to heal and restore physical functioning.

The Bible also contains teachings about spiritual healing, wholeness, and restoration, which may be related to physical health and wellness, including the management of palsy. For example, in Matthew 11:28-30, Jesus invites those who are weary and heavy-laden to come to Him for rest and refreshment.

In addition, the Bible teaches about the importance of compassion, care, and support for individuals with physical disabilities and illnesses, which may be related to palsy. For example, in Matthew 25:36, Jesus teaches that visiting the sick and caring for their needs is a fundamental aspect of loving one's neighbor as oneself.

In conclusion, while the Bible does not specifically address palsy as a modern medical diagnosis, it contains accounts of individuals with symptoms and conditions that may be related to palsy, as well as teachings about spiritual healing, compassion, and care for the physical body. These accounts offer insights into the physical and spiritual aspects of human experience and emphasize the importance of care, support, and understanding for individuals with physical disabilities and illnesses.

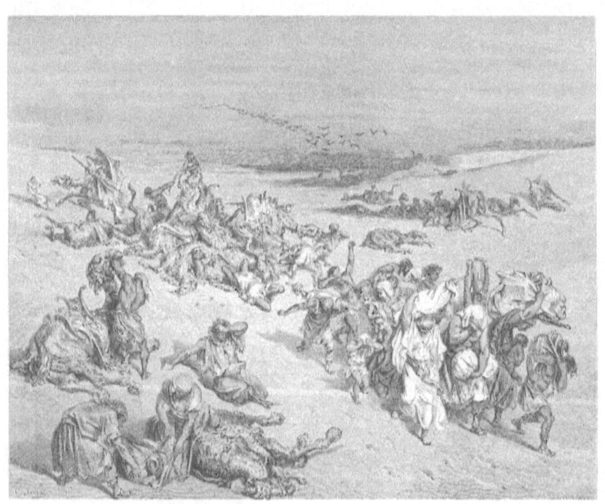

5. Biblical Phytology

Exploring the Healing Plants of the Bible

The Bible contains numerous references to plants and herbs used for medicinal purposes, showcasing the ancient Israelite's knowledge of botany and natural remedies. These biblical medicinal plants were used to treat various ailments, from common colds and fevers to skin conditions and wounds. Many of these plants are still used today in traditional medicine, and some have even been incorporated into modern pharmacology.

The use of biblical medicinal plants is a testament to the ancient Israelite's understanding of the natural world and their resourcefulness in using available resources for healing. This knowledge has been passed down through generations, and many of these plants continue to be used in traditional medicine today.

In this exploration of biblical medicinal plants, we'll delve deeper into the scripture, about these natural medicinal plants, uncovering the wisdom and knowledge of our ancestors.

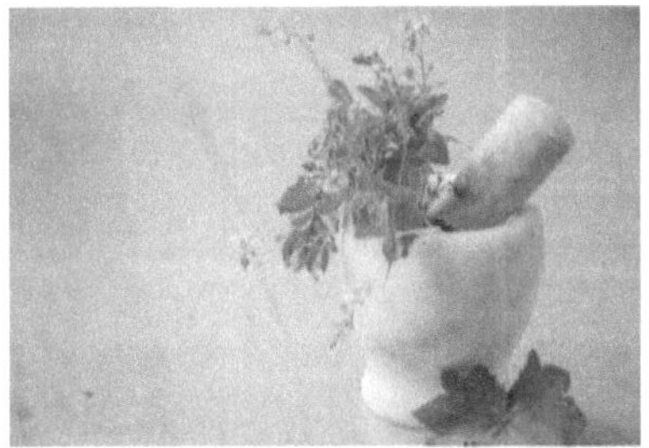

Balm of Gilead (Commiphora Gileadensis)

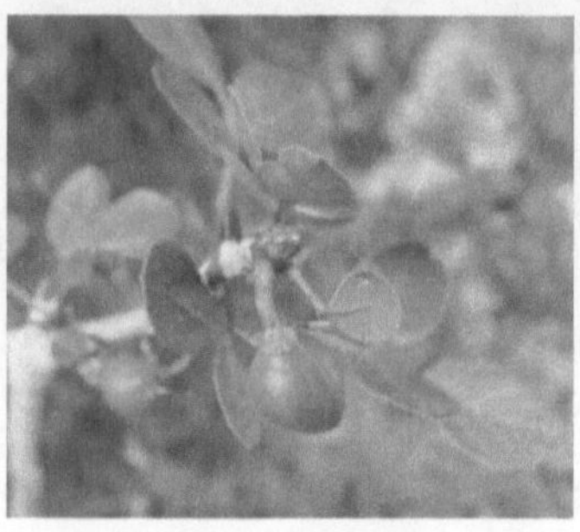

The Balm of Gilead, mentioned in the Bible (Genesis 37:25, Jeremiah 8:22, and 46:11), has been a topic of interest for centuries. This resin, extracted from the *Commiphora opobalsamum* tree, native to the Middle East, was highly valued for its medicinal properties. In the ancient world, it was used to treat various ailments, from wounds and skin conditions to respiratory issues and even emotional distress.

In the Bible, the Balm of Gilead is first mentioned in Genesis 37:25, where a caravan carrying the balm passes by Joseph's brothers as they contemplate selling him into slavery. This reference highlights the balm's value and widespread trade. Later, in Jeremiah 8:22, the prophet laments the absence of the balm, symbolizing the spiritual and physical suffering of God's people. In Jeremiah 46:11, the balm is mentioned as a treatment for the wounds of the nations.

Similar to Jeremiah's time, the people in the New Testament were also wayward. The same people who praised Jesus and covered His path with palm branches on Palm Sunday cried "Crucify Him" a week later on Good Friday. His blood on the cross and willingness to give Himself as a whole for us echoes that of a healing balm that could heal us from our sin. During each Good Friday, we remember that Christ offered and scarified him for us on the cross, reflecting him as the only healing balm who could save our lives and forgive our sins.

The medicinal uses of Balm of Gilead were diverse. Its antiseptic and anti-inflammatory properties made it effective in treating wounds, cuts, and skin conditions like eczema and acne. It was also used to soothe respiratory issues like bronchitis, asthma, and coughs. Additionally, the balm was believed to have calming effects, helping with anxiety, stress, and even emotional pain.

The balm was known to be used in combination with other ingredients such as licorice and honey to increase its potency for solving chest congestion, lard for bruising, swelling, and damage to the skin. Inflammation is what the balm of Gilead is used mostly for. Presently, used also for sunburns and arthritis. Ancient philosophers say that King Solomon was gifted with the balm by Queen Sheba.

The place of Gilead is recognized in the Bible for being the birthplace of the prophet Elijah, the last place where Jacob and Laban met, and the battlefield of Gideon. So, it makes sense that a balm from Gilead would be of great significance in the Bible.

The significance of Balm of Gilead extends beyond its medicinal properties. It symbolized hope, healing, and restoration. In the Bible, it represented God's presence and care, reminding His people of His desire to heal their physical and spiritual wounds.

The Balm of Gilead played a significant role in ancient medicine and biblical symbolism. Its medicinal uses and spiritual significance continue to fascinate scholars and inspire reflection on God's provision and care.

Fig (Ficus Carica)

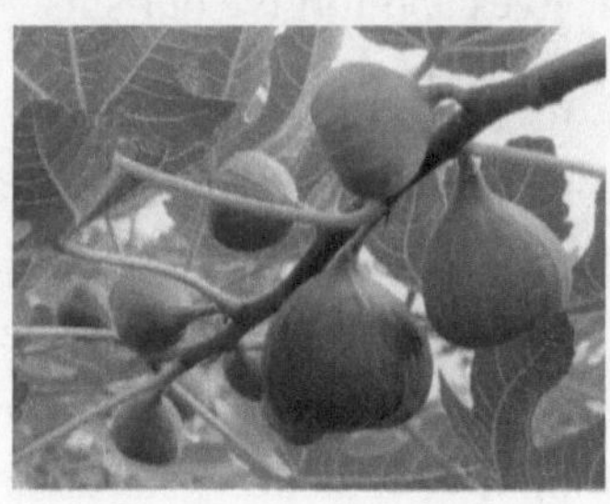

The fig tree is often used as a barograph of the attitude and health of the Israelites. Full, lively, fruitful fig trees are symbols of a healthy and faithful people. Empty, sick fig trees are symbols of suffering and sinful people.

The fig tree, mentioned numerous times in the Bible (Matthew 21:18-20, Mark 11:12-14, Luke 13:6-9), holds significant cultural, spiritual, and medicinal value. In ancient times, figs were not only a staple food but also a trusted remedy for various ailments. The Bible references the medicinal use of figs, highlighting their importance in ancient medicine.

In the Old Testament, figs were used to treat boils and skin conditions (II Kings 20:7, Isaiah 38:21). The fig's sap, rich in antioxidants and anti-inflammatory compounds, was applied topically to soothe and heal skin irritations. Figs were also consumed to aid digestion, relieve constipation, and even treat respiratory issues like bronchitis and coughs.

Hezekiah was sick and near death. And Isaiah the prophet, the son of Amoz, went to him and said to him, "Thus says the Lord: 'Set your house in order, for you shall die and not live'" (Isaiah 38:1). But King Hezekiah prayed gravely to the Lord. He said, "Remember now, O Lord, I pray, how I have walked before you in truth and with a loyal heart, and have done what is good in your sight." As mentioned in Isaiah 38:1, 21 and 2 Kings 20:7,

The Lord answered Hezekiah's prayer and sent the following message, "Let them take a lump of figs, and apply it as a poultice on the boil, and he shall recover". Being suffering from a deadly illness, King Hezekiah might have objected at this simple treatment

Perhaps, the infection had spread and was life threatening. The illness had gone to a scenario where no ordinary treatment could cure. The king felt that God should do some miraculous act to save his life.

But when the command was given to apply a simple natural remedial substance, on following the instructions very carefully, the king was healed.

There is a moral in this story for us to learn. This case demonstrates that divine healing does not diminish the use of natural remedies. The use of such treatments does not reveal the lack of faith. On contrary, a refusal to do so shows, a lack of good judgment.

The Lord might have healed Hezekiah without the use of this fig poultice, but where natural remedies are available; the Lord desires that they should be used in the healing of disease. Therefore, it is our privilege to in-cooperate natural methods, after offering a prayer, to bring about healing from suffering and to help stop the spread of illness.

In the New Testament, Jesus' encounter with the fig tree (Matthew 21:18-20, Mark 11:12-14) symbolizes His power and authority. However, some scholars interpret this episode as a reference to the medicinal use of figs. Jesus' cursing of the fig tree, which withered and died, may represent His condemnation of the religious leaders' lack of spiritual fruitfulness, as well as the unfruitful use of figs for medicinal purposes without acknowledging God's provision.

Figs contain fiber, potassium, and antioxidants, making them a nutritious fruit with various health benefits. They support healthy digestion, lower blood pressure, and even help manage blood sugar levels. The fig's medicinal properties align with biblical accounts of its use in ancient medicine.

The significance of figs extends beyond their medicinal value. In biblical symbolism, figs represent peace, prosperity, and spiritual growth (I Kings 4:25, Micah 4:4, Zechariah 3:10). The fig tree's ability to produce two crops of figs annually made it a symbol of God's abundance and provision.

The medicinal use of figs in the Bible showcases their importance in ancient medicine and spiritual symbolism. As a natural remedy and symbol of God's provision, figs continue to inspire appreciation for nature's gifts and the Bible's timeless wisdom.

Hyssop (Origanum Syriacum)

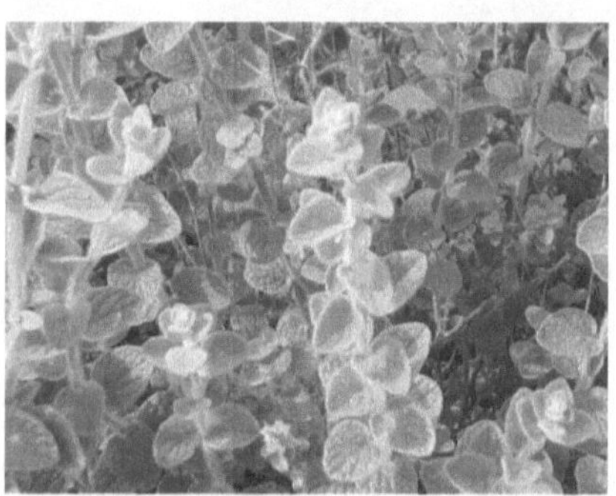

Hyssop, a plant mentioned in the Bible (Exodus 12:22, Leviticus 14:4-6, Psalm 51:7), has been used for centuries for its medicinal properties. In ancient times, hyssop was valued for its antiseptic, anti-inflammatory, and expectant qualities, making it a trusted remedy for various ailments.

In the Old Testament, hyssop was used to purify and cleanse. During the Passover, hyssop was used to apply the lamb's blood to doorposts (Exodus 12:22). Exodus 12:22 says, "Take a bunch of hyssop, dip it into the blood in the basin and put some of the blood on the top and on both sides of the doorframe. None of you shall go out of the door of your house until morning."

This command came from the Lord as the Jewish nation waited to be delivered out of Egypt. God had already brought down nine plagues on Egypt to show His power, but Pharaoh continued to refuse to let God's people leave (Exodus 1-11).

The final plague was the worst of all –God striked down all the firstborns of Egypt, from royal princes to cattle. But He had a plan to protect His people from the disaster about to come. The Israelites were commanded to sacrifice a lamb, one for each family, and to cook and eat the meat. Hyssop was used as a sort of paintbrush to apply the lamb's blood across the doorway of each home.

In Levitical law, hyssop was employed in purification rituals for lepers and those who came into contact with the dead (Leviticus 14:4-6). This symbolic use of hyssop represented spiritual cleansing and forgiveness.

Leviticus 14:4 - "The priest shall order that two live clean birds and some cedar wood, scarlet yarn and hyssop be brought for the person to be cleansed."

Leviticus 14:52 - "He shall purify the house with the bird's blood, the fresh water, the live bird, the cedar wood, the hyssop and the scarlet yarn.

God wanted the Israelite nation to live according to His directions. In return for their obedience, He would provide all that they needed and bless them. One of the ways by which He showed His favor was by healing diseases among the people. He expected them to respond by offering an animal sacrifice as a means of thanksgiving.

A priest used Hyssop, cedar wood, scarlet yarn and a live bird as ingredients to sprinkle blood over someone who'd been healed of a skin disease like leprosy. It was a ceremonial act of cleansing. Likewise, priests also used hyssop in some purification rites.

Hyssop's medicinal properties align with its biblical uses. Its essential oils contain compounds with antiseptic and anti-inflammatory effects, making it effective against infections and respiratory issues like bronchitis and coughs. Hyssop tea has been used to soothe sore throats and calm anxiety.

Psalm 51:7, "Purge me with hyssop, and I shall be clean: wash me, and I shall be whiter than snow," highlights hyssop's symbolic and medicinal significance. This elucidates Hyssop's cleansing effects on the body, mind, and soul. It is a fascinating herb with an affinity for nearly every part of the body. King David's plea for spiritual cleansing and forgiveness is mirrored in hyssop's physical use as a purifying agent.

Hyssop's use in ancient Greek medicine is recorded by Dioscorides and Galen. The plant's properties include expectorant, helping to expel mucus and phlegm. It is used in treating fever, indigestion, and even snakebites. The symbolic connection between hyssop and the Holy Spirit, as mentioned in John 19:29-30

The medicinal use of hyssop in the Bible showcases its importance in ancient medicine and spiritual symbolism. As a natural remedy and symbol of spiritual cleansing, hyssop continues to inspire appreciation for nature's gifts and the Bible's timeless wisdom.

Mandrake (Mandragora Officinarum)

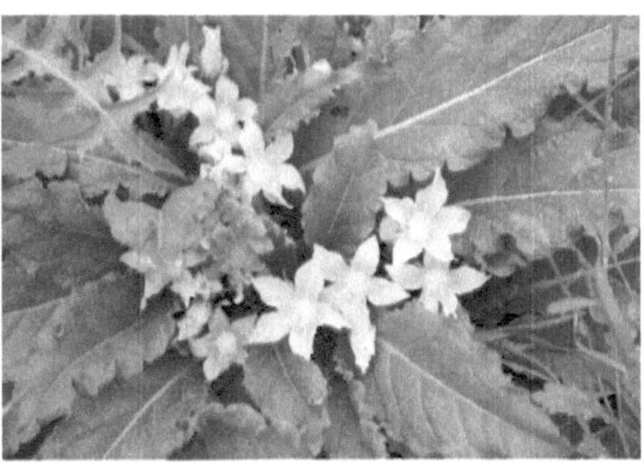

A mandrake is a short-stemmed, flowering plant belonging to the nightshade family. Mandrakes have unusually large, forked root that is similar to the human body with open arms and legs. In the antique world, mandrake roots were commonly prepared and eaten as a fertility drug. There are many references to mandrakes in folklore and delusions in various cultures.

The Mandrake plant, mentioned in the Bible (Genesis 30:14-16, Song of Solomon 7:13), has been used for centuries for its medicinal properties. In ancient times, Mandrake was valued for its sedative, anti-inflammatory, and antiseptic qualities, making it a trusted remedy for various ailments.

In the Old Testament, Rachel uses Mandrake to conceive (Genesis 30:14-16), highlighting its association with fertility and childbirth. Here, Jacob's two wives, Rachel and Leah, struggle for Jacob's attention. Rachel wants a child, and Leah wants more children. Leah's son Reuben found mandrakes in the field and gave them to his mother. Reuben's recognition of the mandrake is particularly significant because it indicates a high level of familiarity with the plant, suggesting he knew its purpose and could distinguish it from other plants or even weeds. Leah traded the mandrakes to Rachel in exchange for the opportunity to sleep with Jacob that night (Genesis 30:14–16). Rachel, who was childless, accepts the trade, believing that the mandrakes would help her conceive at a later time. Leah sleeps with Jacob that night and becomes pregnant with her fifth son (Genesis 30:17). The plant's roots contain alkaloids that can stimulate the uterus and relieve menstrual cramps, making it a natural aid for women's health issues.

Mandrake's medicinal properties align with its biblical uses. Its roots and leaves have been used to treat insomnia, anxiety, and pain. The plant's antiseptic properties make it effective against infections, while its anti-inflammatory properties soothe wounds and reduce swelling.

In the Song of Solomon (7:13), Mandrake is mentioned as a symbol of love and fertility, reinforcing its connection to women's health and childbirth. In the Song of Solomon 7:13 we recite, "The mandrakes send out their fragrance, and at our door is every delicacy, both new and old, that I have stored up for you, my beloved."

The indication of mandrakes in the Song of Solomon is part of a romantic happenstance between Solomon and his new wife. Mandrakes were around them in the countryside, along with grapes, pomegranates, and "every delicacy" (Song of Solomon 7:13). The entire description in verses 10–13 is of a romantic setting that boosts the desire of the husband and wife for each other.

In that scene, the Shulammite invites King Solomon to join her for a sexual rendezvous out of doors in the early morning. "Let us go early to the vineyards to see if the vines have budded, if their blossoms have opened, and if the pomegranates are in bloom - there I will give you my love" (Song of Solomon 7:12). The depiction of this romantic time is full of beautiful imagery, including the mention of mandrakes in the verses that follow, as both husband and wife enjoy each other among the vineyards.

Mandrakes are used in ancient Greek medicine, as recorded by Dioscorides and Galen. Its properties include natural pain reliever and sedative. It is used in treating respiratory issues like bronchitis and asthma.

The medicinal use of Mandrake in the Bible showcases its importance in ancient medicine and spiritual symbolism. As a natural remedy and symbol of fertility and love, Mandrake continues to inspire appreciation for nature's gifts and the Bible's timeless wisdom.

Nard (Nardostachys Jatamansi)

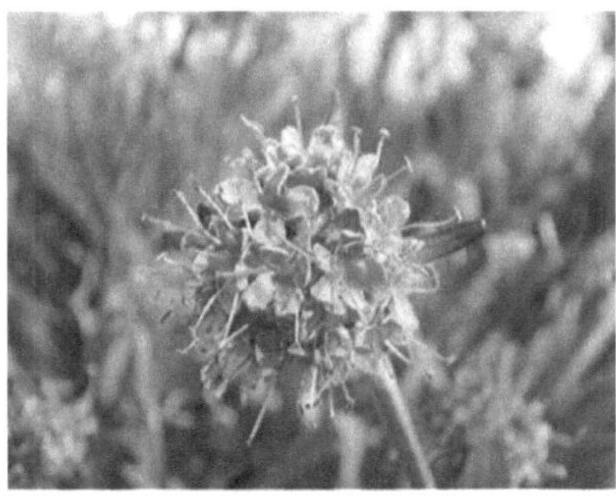

Spikenard is referred in the Bible as "Nard" and is denoted to be used as an ointment and oil. The pure Nard oil was renowned for its pleasant fragrance, and is noted in the Bible to be expensive.

Nardostachys jatamansi is the botanical name of nard mentioned in the Bible. In biblical times, it was considered as valuable and fragrant oil, often used in perfumes and ointments. It was also used in religious ceremonies as a symbol of honor and distinction.

It is a flowering herb found in the Himalayan region at altitudes of 3000–5000 meters. The plant grows to a height of one meter and bear bell-shaped pink flowers. The collection and harvesting of N. jatamansi are done before the first snow, usually from May to July. The rhizomes are crushed and distilled to yield long-lasting amber-colored aromatic oil used in incense, perfume, and herbal medicine. The essential oil has a green, moderately powerful, medicinal, and herbaceous top node that is spicy and sweet. Spikenard essential oil blends well with pine, lavender, patchouli, and vetiver oil. The oil is non-toxic and non-irritating on the skin. It is often used in combination with other short-lived scents like rose. Roots and rhizomes contain a variety of sesquiterpenes and coumarins.

In ancient Greece and Rome, spikenard was used to make a popular ointment called nardinium, which helped to meditate and calm the nerves. When mixed with olive oil, it was used for consecration, dedication, and worship, a continued practice. It was also an ingredient in the Jewish Ketoret incense. As previously mentioned, incense was burned in Jewish temples to mask the smell of animal sacrifices. Traditionally, spikenard and other incense were also used to anoint visitors' foreheads and feet, often covered in dirt from traveling.

Nard, mentioned in the Bible (Song of Solomon 1:12, Mark 14:3, John 12:3), has been used for centuries for its medicinal properties. In ancient times, Nard was valued for its antiseptic, anti-inflammatory, and sedative qualities, making it a trusted remedy for various ailments.

In the Old Testament, Nard is mentioned as a perfume and incense (Song of Solomon 1:12), highlighting its aromatic properties. The plant's essential oils contain compounds with antiseptic and anti-inflammatory effects, making it effective against infections and skin conditions.

In the book of Isaiah, nard is also mentioned in a list of luxurious goods that would be brought to the King of Tyre: "The ships of Tarshish will bring your sons from far away, their silver and gold with them, for the honor of the Lord your God, the Holy One of Israel, who has richly blessed you." (Isaiah 60:9)

In the Old Testament, the nard is seen as a symbol of luxury, richness, and divine honor.

In the New Testament, Nard is famously used by Mary to anoint Jesus' feet (Mark 14:3, John 12:3), symbolizing His upcoming death and burial. This act also showcases Nard's medicinal use, as it would have helped to soothe and calm Jesus' skin. In this context, the nard symbolizes love and devotion, and the anointing demonstrates Mary's devotion to Jesus.

Nard's medicinal properties align with its biblical uses. Its roots and leaves have been used to treat insomnia, anxiety, and pain. The plant's antiseptic properties make it effective against infections, while its anti-inflammatory properties soothe wounds and reduce swelling.

The medicinal use of Nard in the Bible showcases its importance in ancient medicine and spiritual symbolism. As a natural remedy and symbol of devotion and love, Nard continues to inspire appreciation for nature's gifts and the Bible's timeless wisdom.

6. Medical Missionaries

God's Instruments of Healing

Medical missionaries are Christian missionaries who travel to different parts of the world to administer medical treatment and care to those in need, especially in developing countries.

The concept of medical missionaries has its roots in the New Testament, where Jesus Christ commands his disciples to heal the sick and serve the poor. The first Protestant medical missionary was Peter Parker, who was sent to China in 1834 by the American Board of Commissioners for Foreign Missions. The Edinburgh Medical Missionary Society was established in 1841, which became the first medical mission society in Europe.

Medical missionaries work in various parts of the world, providing medical care and medical supplies, clothing, and food to those in need. They also work to prevent the spread of diseases, provide health education, and respond to emergencies and disasters. Some medical missionaries also work to combat human trafficking and provide support to victims of trafficking.

Medical missionaries brought healthcare services to remote, impoverished, or disaster-stricken areas, demonstrating God's love and care. Through their work, they shared the message of God's love, hope, and redemption, often in areas where the Gospel is not well-known.

Dame Edith Mary Brown

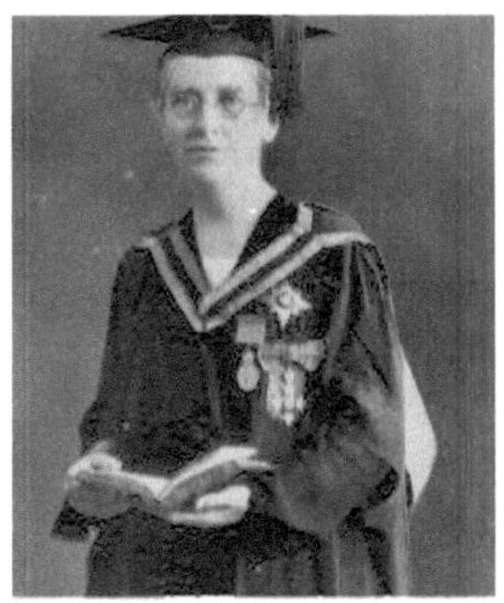

Dame Edith Mary Brown was an English doctor and medical educator. She founded the Christian Medical College Ludhiana in 1894, the first medical training facility for women in Asia, and served as principal of the college for half a century. Brown was a pioneer in the instruction of Indian female doctors and midwives with modern western methods.

Early Life and Education

Brown was born on 24 March 1864 in Whitehaven, Cumberland, England, to George Wightman Brown, a bank manager, and his second wife, Mary. She was the second daughter born to Mary.

Brown began her education at Manchester High School for Girls before moving to Croydon High School, an all-girls independent school in London. Having won a scholarship, she studied natural sciences at Gorton College, Cambridge. She took second class honors in 1885.

An elder sister was a missionary, which developed in her an interest in medicine and missionary work. She began her profession as science teacher at Exeter High School for Girls, before being provided with financial aid by the Baptist Mission

Society to study medicine. She then entered the London School of Medicine for Women, and went on to graduate with the Scottish Triple Qualification in 1891; the Licentiate of the Royal College of Physicians of Edinburgh, the Licentiate of the Royal College of Surgeons of Edinburgh, and the Licentiate of the Royal College of Physicians and Surgeons of Glasgow.

Career and Missionary Work

Accepting the request of The Baptist Missionary Society, she arrived Bombay on 9 November 1891. She was stunned by the medical conditions in India and felt a need to educate women and midwives.

Brown set out on her own after two years serving with various missions,. In January 1894, a woman in Bristol donated 50 dollars to rent her with an old schoolhouse in Ludhiana, Punjab. She organized a Christian medical training center for women, the North India School of Medicine for Christian Women, starting with four students and four faculties.

The first medical school for women in India grew into a full college with medical, nursing and pharmacy schools, and a hospital with 200 beds. The college was supported by grants from the Punjab government, as well as women's auxiliaries in London, Edinburgh, Glasgow, Australia, Canada, the United States and New Zealand. Since 1909, it had opened its doors to non-Christians. The school was renamed as Christian Medical College, Ludhiana in 1911.

Punjab was split between India and Pakistan during the partition of British India in 1947, resulting in massacres of thousands in Ludhiana. Inspite of violence, the college and hospital remained safe from attack. The hospital became an emergency center for the seriously injured.

In November 1951, on the 50th anniversary of Brown's arrival to India, the college had graduated 411 doctors, 143 nurses, 168 pharmacy dispensers and more than 1,000 midwives. Brown retired as principal in 1952 and moved to Kashmir.

Dame Hood and Death

In the 1932 New Year Honors, Brown was made a Dame Commander of the Order of the British Empire. At the age of 92, Brown died on 6 December 1956 in Srinagar, India.

Henry Martyn Scudder

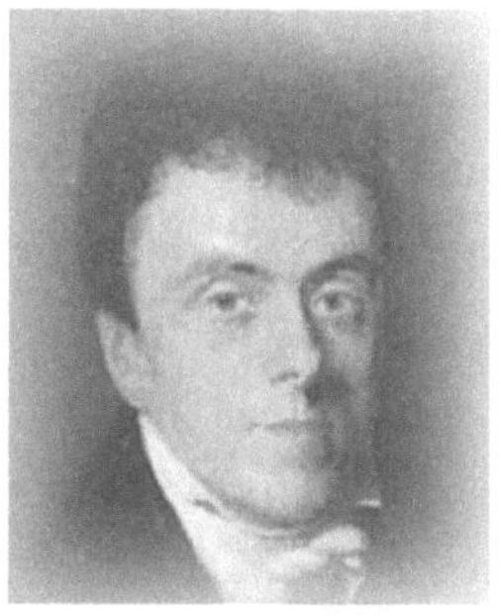

Henry Martyn Scudder was a missionary under the American Board of Commissioners for Foreign Missions and Board of Foreign Missions of the Reformed Church in America to Japan and South India—to the American Madura Mission and American Madras Mission. He also established the American Arcot Mission, North Arcot of South India under the Madras Presidency.

He was born at Panditeripo, Ceylon, on 5 February 1822. He was the eldest son of John Scudder Sr., the first American medical missionary to India and second missionary to American Madras Mission at Madras. Sr. Scudder arrived at Madras in September 1836, after East India Company opened India in 1833 to missionaries of all lands, including non-British missionaries. He joined his father as a missionary at Madras in 1844.

in 1832, He went to the United States, and graduated at the University of the City of New York in 1840 and Union Theological Seminary. He was ordained by American Board of Commissioners for Foreign Missions (ABCFM) in 1843. The following year he was sent as an ABCFM missionary to Madura, India, where he served from 1844 to 1846 and in 1846 to Madras, where he worked until 1850. After his arrival to Madras from United States, he studied medicine at Madras Medical College. Later, he received his M.D degree from New York University. In 1850, Henry Scudder visited the neighboring districts of Arcot and found that millions of souls never heard of Jesus Christ. Hence, he obtained the permission from British Raj to make the city of Arcot as the center of a new mission in the northern districts of Arcot. The father and son opened a mission in the Arcot district, as a chief station of North Arcot Mission. The mission introduced Western medical science among the natives Tamil population of the districts. The British Madras Government of Madras Presidency gave him a building, sufficient land for the construction of hospital, and contributed its expenses. Initially, when no house was available for residence, he took a rented house at Wallajanagar and opened a dispensary with the purpose of winning a favorable entrance for the gospel. At once, nine children and nine grandchildren were associated with that mission. He was among the Scudders in India who dedicated more than 1,100 combined years to the Christian medical mission service by 42 members of four generations in the family.

He published numerous books in Sanskrit, Tamil, and Telugu. With excellent proficiency in Tamil language, he published Spiritual Teaching, The Bazaar Book, and Jewel Mine of

Salvation that had become valuable aid to missionaries and native preachers. He also made the translation of liturgy into Tamil.

In 1864, as his health was poor, he returned to America, and he became a pastor of a church in San Francisco. He held pastorates at New Jersey, New York and Chicago. He built churches in Brooklyn and Chicago, and engaged in pastoral work for around 20 years. From 1887 to 1889 he was in the mission field in Japan. He died on 4 June 1895 in Winchester, Massachusetts.

Ida Sophia Scudder

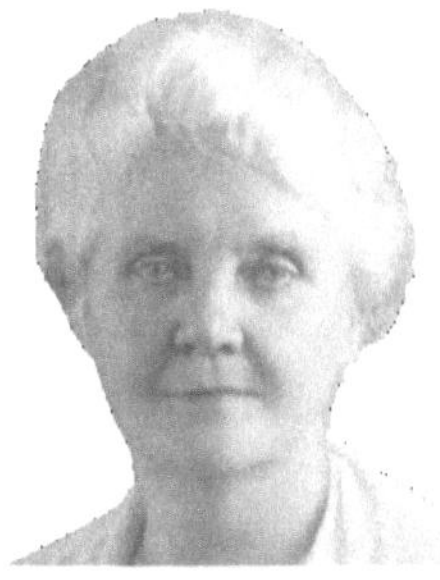

Ida Sophia Scudder was a third-generation American medical missionary in India. She sought to improve the plight of Indian women by fighting against plague, cholera and leprosy was born to John Scudder and Sophia on December 9, 1870 (née Weld), part of a line of medical missionaries that started with her grandfather, John Scudder Sr. They were members of the Reformed Church in America. Growing up as a child in India, she witnessed famine, poverty and disease. She was invited to study at Northfield Seminary in Massachusetts. In 1890, she returned to India to help her father when her mother was ailing at the mission bungalow at Tindivanam. During her stay, she witnessed three women died in childbirth in one night.

Scudder graduated from Cornell Medical College, New York City in 1899. She then headed back to India and started a tiny medical dispensary and clinic for women at Vellore. Her father died in 1900, soon after she arrived in India. In two years, she treated 5,000 patients.

Scudder opened the Mary Taber Schell Hospital in 1902. She decided to open a medical school for girls only and received 151 applications the first year in 1918. In 1928, ground was captured for the medical school campus on 200 acres at Bagayam, Vellore. In 1928, Mahatma Gandhi visited the medical school. Scudder traveled a number of times to the United States to raise funds for the college and hospital. In 1945, the college was opened to men as well. In 2003 the Vellore Christian Medical Center was the largest Christian hospital in the world, with 2000 beds, and its medical school is now one of the premier medical colleges in India. In 2023, the center was ranked number 3 college by the National Institute Ranking Framework (NIRF). The Center was later headed by Scudder's niece, Ida Belle Scudder.

In 1952, Scudder received the Elizabeth Blackwell Citation from the New York Eye and Ear Infirmary, as one of 1952's five outstanding women doctors. She died on May 23, 1960 at her bungalow. In 1960, Rajendra Prasad, then President of India, quoted Scudder as a "great lady, whose dedication and planned working are exemplary". The Ida Scudder School in Viruthampet, Vellore, is named in her honor. A commemorative stamp was released by the Department of Posts on August 12, 2000, as part of the centenary celebrations of the Christian Medical College. The First-day cover portrays Dr Ida Scudder.

William James Wanless

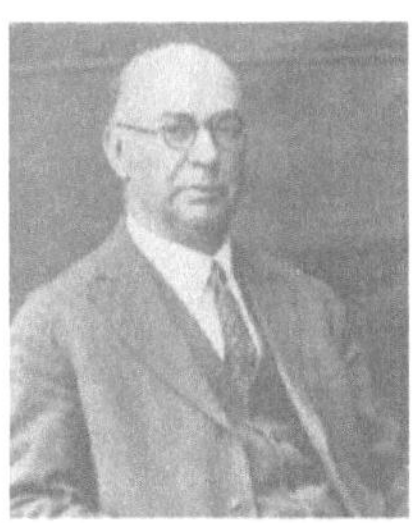

Early Life and Education

William James Wanless was born on May 1, 1865, to Elizabeth and John Wanless in the then-community of Charleston, Province of Canada. He was the sixth of 14 children, including two elder brothers who died in childhood. His father, born in Barrow, Alwinton, and Northumberland, England on December 30, 1832, immigrated to the United States with his family at the age of 17.

He graduated from the New York University School of Medicine in 1889. He married Mary Elizabeth Marshall on September 5, 1889, in Canada, and sailed for India the same year. Mary gave birth to Ethel at Miraj on Dec 2, 1891. Mary died on August 12, 1906. On December 5, 1907, Dr William married again at Kodoli to Lillian Emery Havens, who survived him. Lillian gave birth to 3 children: Harold L. Wanless, Robert Emery Wanless, and Margaret Elizabeth Wanless.

Wanless was a delegate to the 1910 World Missionary Conference held in Edinburgh, Scotland, and was president of the Missionary Medical Association of India from 1911 to 1928. In 1918 he was made a Fellow of the American College of Surgeons. He was erroneously reported as dead in 1922; the incorrect report and its subsequent retraction made headlines in the United States.

Mission in India

The Bryn Mawr Presbyterian Church, of Bryn Mawr, Pennsylvania, sent Dr. Wanless to India in 1889. In 1891, he selected the rustic town of Miraj in Maharashtra State for the mission hospital. The Mission was started as a one-room dispensary in a very small rented place at a busy bazaar, and he was assisted by his wife, Mary, a trained nurse. The Rajah of Miraj, Rajah Sir Gangadharrao Ganesh (Bala Saheb) Patwardhan, provided him with land for a hospital which was formally opened in 1894, in a part of the city now known as Wanlesswadi.

With the establishment of a hospital, the need for higher quality medical care was increasingly felt, and towards that end a School of Nursing was founded in 1897 under the superintendence of Miss Elizabeth Foster. It has since steadily developed into one of the best nursing schools in Maharashtra.

The Mary Wanless Hospital was founded in memory of Wanless's first wife Mary after her death in 1906. Now called the Mary Wanless Hospital / Miraj Medical Centre, it still attracts hundreds of poor and needy patients from across India and abroad. He established the Miraj Christian Medical School in 1907, which later graduated its first group of 17 students, with its only qualified teacher being Wanless himself. In 1917 the medical school was recognized for a Diploma of Licentiate by the College of Physicians and Surgeons of Mumbai (LCPS), similar to the LRCP of the Royal College of Surgeons (MRCS) of England.

Wanless established a Tuberculosis Sanatorium in 1920. At the time of his retirement in 1928, money was raised by citizens and his friends to erect a new building called the Wanless Tuberculosis Sanatorium, now known as Wanless Chest Hospital. It is one of the premier institutions in the country.

Retirement and Legacy

In 1928, after almost forty years of medical missionary service in India, Wanless retired to live in the United States. He wrote a book, Medicine in India, on his life as a doctor in India. He died at his home, 1016 Matillja Street, Glendale, California, on March 3, 1933, and was buried at Forest Lawn Memorial Park in the same city. His wife Lillian died in 1973 at the age of 99 at their home in Glendale, California. Wanless's son Harold later carried on his father's tradition by studying medicine at the University of Toronto.

Since its inception over 115 years ago his medical mission has grown into an institution consisting of a 550-bed teaching hospital affiliated with India's Government Medical College, a College of Nursing, an Institute of Pharmacy and various paramedical programs.

The Wanless Hospital and Wanless Chest Hospital are now located in the township of 'Wanlesswadi', that is 'Wanless town', made notable for its medical institutions. The name was given it by its citizens in that part of India and is recognized by the federal government of India. Wanlesswadi has its own Postal Index Number, 416414, and the Indian Railways also has a station named 'Wanlesswadi' on its Miraj–Sangli Route, which opened on April 1, 1907, for the use by ill or needy patients from across India and from abroad.

As a secondary and tertiary care center, Wanless Hospital serves a large part of western Maharashtra and North Karnataka. The Wanless Hospital reputedly provides the best possible medical care to all its patients; an institution for comprehensive and dedicated health care.

Honours

The badge of a Knight Bachelor. He first received the silver Kaisar-i-Hind (Emperor in India) medal of second class in 1912. He received the order of gold medal of first class in 1920, in recognition of his philanthropic and humanitarian work for India. The third honor was bestowed upon him on January 2, 1928, by His Majesty, George V of the United Kingdom, was a knighthood of the British Empire, conferring upon him the degree and honor.

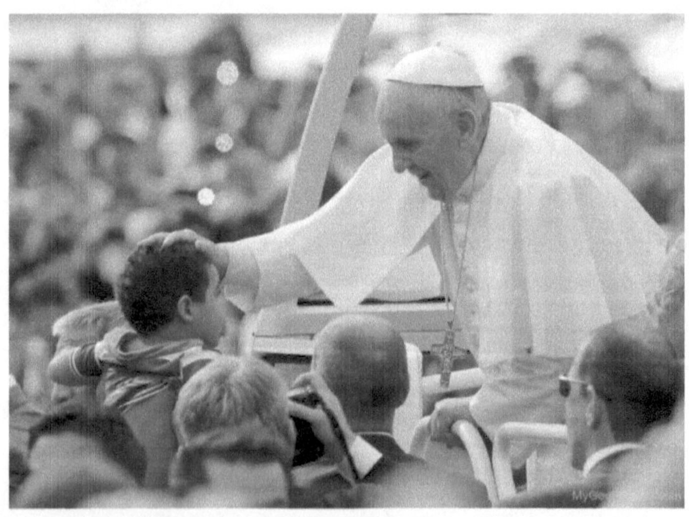

7. The Saintly Healers

Inspiring Lives of Patron Saints of Healthcare

Saints of healthcare are revered for their contributions to the field of medicine and healing. Some notable saints of healthcare include:

- **Saint Raphael the Archangel:** Patron of healers and the blind.

- **Saint Luke the Evangelist:** Patron of doctors.

- **Saint Agatha:** Patroness of nurses and those with breast cancer.

- **Saints Cosmas and Damian:** Patron saints of doctors and surgeons.

- **Saint Peregrine:** Patron saint of those who suffer from cancer.

- **Saint John of God:** Patron saint of nurses and hospitals.

- **Saint Camillus of Lellis:** Patron of hospitals and hospital workers.

- **Saint Rene Goupil:** Patron of anesthesiologists.

- **Saint Frances Xavier Cabrini:** Patron of orphans and hospital administrators.

- **Saint Gianna Beretta Molla:** Patron of physicians and unborn children.

- **Saint Albert the Great:** Patron saint of scientists and medical technicians.

- **Blessed James Salomone:** Patron of cancer patients.

- **Saint Catherine of Siena:** Patroness of those who care for the sick.

- **Saint Martin de Porres:** Patron of public health workers.

St. Luke the Evangelist

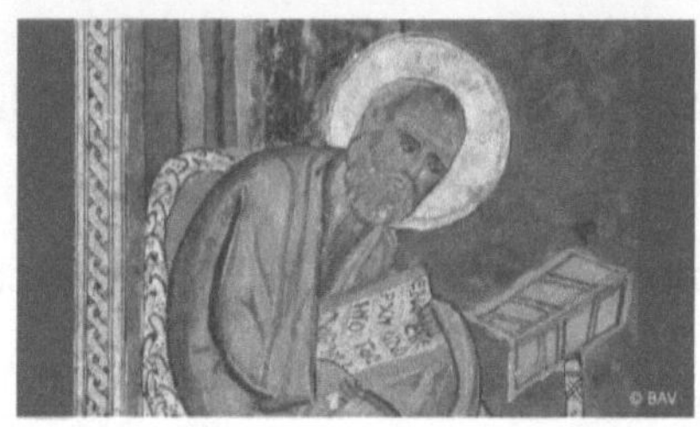

St. Luke the Evangelist is one of the most revered saints in the Catholic Church, and is honored as the patron saint of physicians. As a companion of St. Paul and a skilled physician himself, Luke's contributions to the early Christian Church are immeasurable. His Gospel, which bears his name, is a testament to his faith and dedication to spreading the teachings of Christ. In this essay, we will explore the life and legacy of St. Luke, his role as a physician, and his continued influence on the medical profession.

Life and Legacy

St. Luke was born in Antioch, Syria, in the first century AD. Little is known about his early life, but it is believed that he was a skilled physician and painter. He became a convert to Christianity and joined St. Paul on his missionary journeys, accompanying him to Rome and other parts of the Mediterranean.

St. Luke the Evangelist, also known as St. Luke the Physician, was in fact both a physician and a slave. This was quite common that owners of slaves had someone around to take care of them when they were sick. He was also the author of one of the Gospels and part of the Acts of the Apostles. In his writing, it is said that he used medical terminologies and in describing his care, it reflected what is found in the Hippocratic Oath. From his writings, we can also see that Luke had an attention and care for the poor and the oppressed. He encouraged tenderness and compassion as seen in the stories of Lazarus and the Good Samaritan.

As a physician, Luke was deeply committed to his patients and his faith. He saw his medical practice as a way to serve God and humanity, and his compassion and empathy earned him the respect and admiration of his peers. His Gospel, which is the longest of the four Gospels, is a testament to his faith and his commitment to spreading the teachings of Christ.

Role as Patron Saint of Physicians

St. Luke's role as patron saint of physicians is a natural extension of his life and legacy. His commitment to his patients and his faith, as well as his skill and compassion as a physician, make him an ideal model for medical professionals. His feast day, October 18, is celebrated by physicians and medical professionals around the world, who seek his intercession and guidance.

St. Luke's influence on the medical profession extends beyond his patronage. His Gospel contains several accounts of Jesus' healing miracles, which have inspired countless physicians and medical professionals throughout history. His emphasis on compassion, empathy, and service to others has shaped the ethical and moral principles of the medical profession.

Symbolism and Iconography

In art and iconography, St. Luke is often depicted with a winged ox, which represents his role as a physician and his connection to the Gospel. The ox is also a symbol of strength, endurance, and sacrifice, reflecting Luke's dedication to his patients and his faith.

The colors associated with St. Luke are red and blue, which represent his martyrdom and his heavenly origin. His image is often surrounded by symbols of medicine, such as the caduceus and the staff, which represent his role as a healer and his commitment to serving others.

Devotional Practices

St. Luke is often honored through devotional practices such as prayer, meditation, and the recitation of the Rosary. His intercession is sought by physicians and medical professionals, who ask for his guidance and protection in their work.

Many hospitals and medical institutions are named after St. Luke, and his image is often displayed in medical facilities and clinics. His feast day is celebrated with special masses and ceremonies, which honor his legacy and his contributions to the medical profession.

Miracles and Healings

The impact of Saint Luke's work is felt throughout both the artistic and medical spheres. By incorporating principles of both art and science into his writing, Luke connected the divine to the physical, allowing those professions to flourish.

St. Luke's intercession has been credited with numerous miracles and healings throughout history. Many physicians and medical professionals have reported experiencing his guidance and protection in their work, and have attributed their success to his intercession.

One famous story of St. Luke's intercession is that of a young physician named Giuseppe Moscati, who was struggling to diagnose and treat a patient with a rare and mysterious illness. After praying to St. Luke, Moscati received a vision of the patient's condition and was able to develop an effective treatment. This story, and many others like it, testifies to the power and efficacy of St. Luke's intercession.

St. Luke the Evangelist is a powerful patron saint for physicians and medical professionals, whose intercession and guidance are sought by many. His legacy as a physician, evangelist, and martyr continues to inspire and uplift those who seek his aid, and his feast day is a celebration of God's mercy and love for humanity.

Through his life and legacy, St. Luke reminds us of the importance of compassion, empathy, and service to others. His commitment to his patients and his faith is a model for medical professionals everywhere, and his intercession is a source of comfort and strength for those who seek his aid. His feast is celebrated every year on 18 October.

Raphael the Archangel

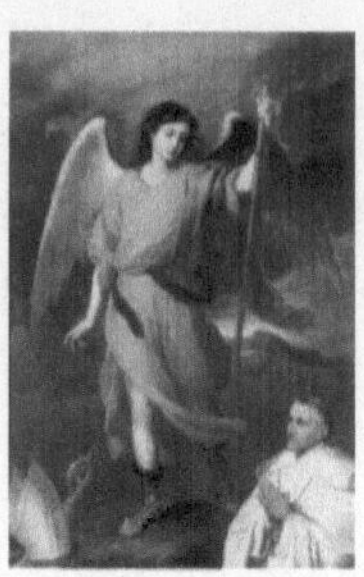

St. Raphael the Archangel is one of the most revered and beloved saints in the Catholic Church. As the patron saint of the sick, he is often invoked for his intercession and guidance by those who are suffering from physical, emotional, or spiritual ailments. His name, which means "God heals," reflects his role as a divine healer and comforter. In this essay, we will explore the life and legacy of St. Raphael, his role as a patron saint, and the many ways in which he continues to inspire and uplift those who seek his aid.

Raphael the Archangel is a shining light of comfort and hope in an often chaotic world. He stepped into his role as patron saint of healing long ago, and today we have much to thank him for. We can reach out to Saint Raphael the Archangel with our prayers, knowing that he will always be beside us throughout our most difficult times. It doesn't matter how desperate our situation may appear, God has provided us with an angel on earth who is ready to listen to our pleas. May we never forget that even when everything else seems lost, Saint Raphael the Archangel is there to bring peace and joy back into our lives.

Raphael was an Archangel with a heart of gold, sent by God to assist humanity in its time of distress. He possessed both wisdom and immense power, but also wielded a compassionate and caring nature.

In the Bible, Raphael is described as the "healing angel".

Devotion to Raphael as a patron of healing also became popular in the Middle Ages, and many hospitals and medical institutions were dedicated to him. Even today, many people invoke his intercession for physical and spiritual healing, and his feast day is celebrated on September 29th.

Life and Legacy

St. Raphael is one of the seven archangels who stand before the throne of God, and is revered as a powerful intercessor and healer. St. Raphael is invoked as the patron saint of the sick because of his role in the Book of Tobit in the Old Testament. In the story, Tobit becomes blind and is advised by his son Tobias to seek the help of a kinsman named Azariah, who is actually St. Raphael in disguise. St. Raphael guides Tobias on a journey to collect a debt owed to Tobit, and along the way, they encounter a demon that had been tormenting a young woman named Sarah. St. Raphael instructs Tobias to catch a fish and use its organs to drive the demon away, which is successful. Later, St. Raphael helps heal Tobit's blindness and reveals his true identity as an angel sent by God to help them. As a result of this story, St. Raphael has been associated with healing and has become a patron saint of the sick.

Throughout his journey with Tobias, Raphael demonstrated his compassion, wisdom, and healing powers. He taught Tobias about the importance of prayer, fasting, and almsgiving, and encouraged him to trust in God's providence. Raphael's guidance and protection helped Tobias navigate the challenges of his journey, and ultimately led him to a deeper understanding of God's love and care.

Through his life and legacy, St. Raphael reminds us of the importance of trusting in God's providence, and of seeking His guidance and protection in times of need. His intercession is a source of comfort and strength for those who are suffering, and his image is a reminder of God's mercy and love for humanity.

Role as Patron Saint

As patron saint of the sick, St. Raphael is often invoked for his intercession and guidance by those who are suffering from physical, emotional, or spiritual ailments. His feast day, September 29, is celebrated by many Christians around the world, who seek his aid and protection.

St. Raphael's role as a healer is not limited to physical ailments, but also extends to spiritual and emotional suffering. He is often called upon to comfort the grieving, strengthen the weak, and guide those who are lost or confused. His intercession is sought by those who are struggling with illness, addiction, or mental health issues, and by those who are seeking comfort and solace in times of sorrow or distress.

Symbolism and Iconography

In art and iconography, St. Raphael is often depicted with a staff and a fish, symbols of his role as a healer and guide. His staff represents his authority and power as a divine messenger, while the fish represents his ability to guide and protect those who are seeking his aid.

The colors associated with St. Raphael are blue and gold, which represent his heavenly origin and his role as a divine messenger. His image is often surrounded by symbols of healing, such as the cross, the crown of thorns, and the lily, which represent his role as a healer and comforter.

Devotional Practices

St. Raphael is often honored through devotional practices such as prayer, meditation, and the recitation of the Rosary. His intercession is sought through the prayer "O Raphael, heavenly physician, we beseech thee, pray for us," which is often recited by those who are seeking his aid.

Many people also seek St. Raphael's intercession through the use of sacramentals, such as holy water, blessed oil, and medals. These sacramentals are believed to possess a special power and efficacy, and are often used to invoke St. Raphael's protection and guidance.

Miracles and Healings

St. Raphael's intercession has been credited with numerous miracles and healings throughout history. Many people have reported being cured of physical and emotional ailments, and have attributed their healing to St. Raphael's intercession.

One famous story of St. Raphael's intercession is that of a young girl named Gemma di Gianni, who was suffering from a severe illness. Her parents invoked St. Raphael's aid, and Gemma was miraculously healed. This story, and many others like it, testifies to the power and efficacy of St. Raphael's intercession.

St. Raphael the Archangel is a powerful patron saint for the sick and suffering, whose intercession and guidance are sought by many. His legacy as a divine healer and comforter continues to inspire and uplift those who seek his aid, and his feast day is a celebration of God's mercy and love for humanity.

As a result, St. Raphael has become a popular saint to invoke for healing, particularly in the Catholic and Orthodox traditions.

Saint Camillus De Lellis

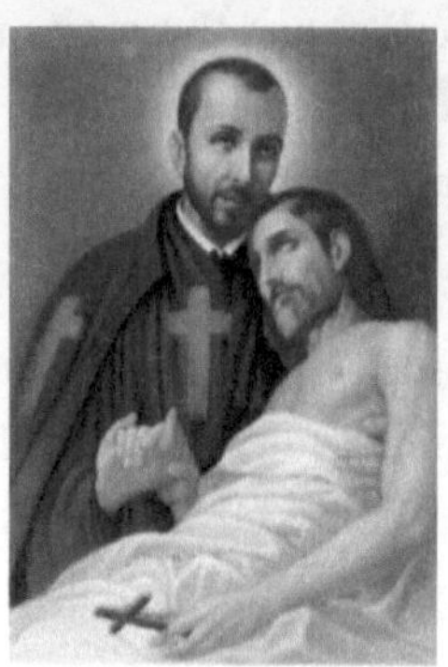

St. Camillus de Lellis is a revered saint in the Catholic Church, known for his tireless dedication to the sick and the poor. As the founder of the Order of the Ministers of the Sick, also known as the Camillians, he is revered as the patron saint of hospitals, nurses, and the sick. His selfless service and compassion towards the suffering have made him a beloved figure in the history of the Church.

Early Life and Conversion

Camillus de Lellis was an Italian nobleman born in 1550 who served as a soldier, fighting the Turks. Three times between 1571 and 1584, his abscessed leg forced him to seek care in a Roman hospital; each time he worked there during and after his treatment. He was disgusted by the bad care in the hospital and decided a religious order devoted to helping the sick was the best way to better physical and spiritual care. In 1585, he founded the

Ministers of the Sick, today called the Order of Saint Camillus. It gained full papal approval as a religious order in 1591. By 1607, it had 242 members working in ten leading Italian cities

He tried to enter the Capuchin novitiate three times, but each time the wound in his leg, coupled with his lack of education, forced him to leave.

He went to Rome and entered the hospital of St. Giacomo, and met St. Phillip Neri, who would become his confessor. Camillus had no way to pay for his hospital stay, so he began ministering to the sick and dying. Through his persistent work, Camillus eventually became superintendent of the hospital.

While at the hospital, he was studying with the Jesuits, and though he still occasionally gambled and fought, he eventually completed his studies for the priesthood and was ordained at age 34, in 1584.

Founding of the Order

Motivated by his work in the hospital, Father Camillus assembled a group of Catholic religious and lay followers to help tend to the needs of suffering patients, calling his group the "Servants of the Sick."

The Servants would be summoned to hospitals, and to prisons and private houses, to tend to the needs of the sick and dying.

In 1586, Pope Sixtus V approved Camillus' group, and in 1591 Pope Gregory XIV confirmed the Servants of the Sick- with the name changed to the 'Order of the Ministers of the Infirm'- as a religious order. Members of the order wear a red cross on their black cassocks and capes, which Camillus reportedly said was to "frighten the devil."

In addition to the traditional vows of poverty, chastity, and obedience, members of the order take a vow of unfailing service to the sick, even at risk to their own lives. The order, today made up of priests and brothers, is often known simply as the "Camillans."

Two congregations of the Camillans for women were created in the 19th century, and secular institutes were established in the 20th century.

Service to the Sick

Camillus's service to the sick was marked by his compassion, empathy, and selflessness. He believed that the sick were not just physical bodies but also spiritual souls, and he sought to minister to both. He introduced innovative methods of care, such as the use of clean linens and the provision of fresh air and water. He also emphasized the importance of prayer and spiritual support for the sick.

Camillus himself was totally devoted to the poor and sick, and though he himself was very ill, he would spend time with the sick even while unable to walk, by crawling from bed to bed to see if the other patients needed help. Upon learning that he himself was incurably ill, Camillus responded: "I rejoice in what has been told me. We shall go into the house of the Lord."

Upon receiving the Eucharist one last time, he said: "O Lord, I confess that I am the most wretched of sinners, most undeserving of thy favor; but save me by thy infinite goodness. My hope is placed in thy divine mercy by thy precious blood."

Camillus died on July 14, 1614. Benedict XIV canonized him in 1746, and in 1886, Leo XIII proclaimed him patron of all hospitals and of the sick.

Pius XI later named him- along with Saint John of God- one of the two main co-patrons of nurses and nursing associations in 1930.

Patronage of Hospitals

Camillus's dedication to the sick and his innovative methods of care have made him the patron saint of hospitals. His feast day, July 14, is celebrated by hospitals and healthcare professionals around the world. His intercession is sought by those who work in healthcare, as well as by those who are sick or suffering.

Symbolism and Iconography

Camillus is often depicted in art and iconography with a red cross on his chest, symbolizing his dedication to the sick and the poor. He is also depicted with a pitcher and a towel, symbolizing his service to the sick and his humility.

Devotional Practices

Camillus is honored through devotional practices such as prayer, meditation, and the recitation of the Rosary. His intercession is sought by those who work in healthcare, as well as by those who are sick or suffering. Many hospitals and healthcare institutions are named after him, and his image is often displayed in hospitals and clinics.

Miracles and Healings

Camillus's intercession has been credited with numerous miracles and healings throughout history. Many people have reported experiencing his guidance and protection in their work, as well as his intercession in times of illness and suffering.

Pope Francis met with men and women religious from the Camillian Charismatic Family in March 2019. He praised those present for their work of "loving and generous donation to the sick, carrying out a precious mission, in the Church and in society, alongside the suffering."

Through fidelity to their founder, and by listening to and accompanying those experiencing poverty and suffering today, the pope said, the Camillians "will know how to make light shine, always new, on the gift received; and many young people the world over will be able to feel attracted by and to join with you, to continue to bear witness to God's tenderness."

St. Camillus de Lellis is a powerful patron saint for hospitals, nurses, and the sick, whose intercession and guidance are sought by many. Through his life and legacy, Camillus reminds us of the importance of charity, humility, and simplicity in serving the sick and the poor. His feast day is a celebration of God's mercy and love for humanity, and his intercession is a source of comfort and strength for those who seek his aid.

Saints Cosmas and Damian

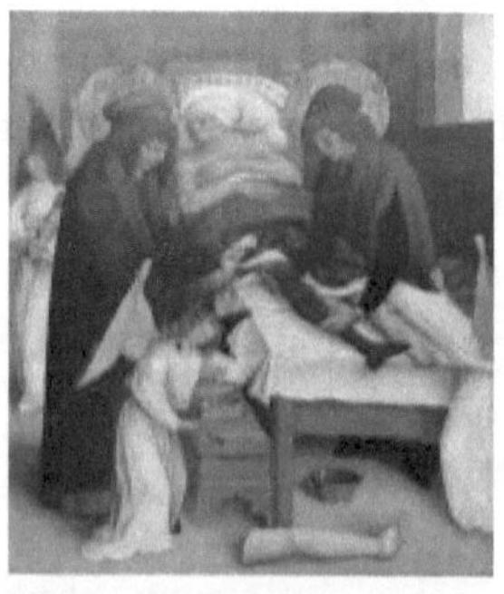

St. Cosmas and Damian are two of the most revered saints in the Catholic Church, known for their unwavering dedication to the sick and the poor. As physicians and martyrs, they are revered as the patron saints of medicine, and their feast day, September 26, is celebrated by healthcare professionals around the world. Their selfless service and compassion towards the suffering have made them beloved figures in the history of the Church.

Early Life and Martyrdom

Cosmas and Damian were Arabian twins, born of devoutly Christian parents around 270 CE. They grew up with three other brothers in Aegeae, a small town between Turkey and Syria and on the route from Antioch to Tarsus, an ancient city in south-central Turkey near the Mediterranean Sea. This region was within the expansive Roman Empire, and the twins lived during the reign of Emperor Diocletian and his local governor, Lysias.

They embraced Christianity and practiced medicine and surgery without a fee. They reputedly cured blindness, fever, paralysis and reportedly expelled a breast serpent. They were arrested by Lysias, governor of Cilicia (modern day Ã‡ukurova, Turkey) during the Diocletian persecution because of their faith and fame as healers. Emperor Diocletian was a religious conservative and favored the traditional Olympian Gods. He issued a series of edicts that condemned the Christians in his attempt to wipe out Christianity from his empire.

Lysias sentenced the twins and their three brothers to death. The family were thrown into the sea but were saved by angels. The authorities then tried burning them at the stake but they remained unharmed. They were then stoned, crucified and shot with arrows but to no effect. They were finally beheaded and their bodies carried to the ancient Syrian city of Cyrrhus, the ruins of which lie very close to Aleppo. A basilica was erected over the tomb of the martyred twins and it became a site of pilgrimage.

Hundreds of healing miracles are attributed to the twin saints. They are most famous for the miracle of the black leg. The story goes that there lived a devout man, who served at the church dedicated to the saints in Rome and had a diseased leg. As he slept, the saints appeared to him carrying an ointment and an instrument. In his dream, the saints decided to remove his diseased leg surgically and grafted a healthy leg from a recently-deceased Ethiopian who was buried in another church. When this man awoke, he reached for his leg and felt no pain. He also apparently reached for a candle and observed that he now had two healthy legs although one was not his! When he was recovered enough, he was able to leap out from his bed and announce the happy news. The Wellcome Library in London holds a beautiful oil painting entitled 'A verger's dream: St. Cosmas and Damian performing a miraculous cure by transplantation of a leg' in their collection and is available to view on request.

The reputation of the saints spread widely through Europe. Emperor Justinian, who reigned from 527-565 AD, believed he was healed by their intercession and dedicated two churches in Constantinople, which was the capital city of the Roman/Byzantine Empire, in gratitude. Relics were dispersed across the continent. Their cult however did not resonate in England with only five churches dedicated to them. Early depictions of the saints did not distinguish which of them was the physician and which the pharmacist. Pharmacists however, identified St. Damian as a patron. The west front of Salisbury Cathedral has statues of the saints in niches 139 and 140. The statue of St. Damian in niche 140, can be identified as the pharmacist saint as he is holding a pestle and mortar in one hand and has the other raised as though to reproach his brother, St. Cosmas. All of the statues above the doors on the west front of the cathedral face the Christ child on St. Christopher's shoulder except St. Cosmas who is positioned facing his brother. This is perhaps to emphasize their

Patronage of Medicine

Cosmas and Damian's dedication to the sick and the poor, as well as their martyrdom, have made them the patron saints of medicine. They are revered by healthcare professionals around the world, who seek their intercession and guidance in their work. Their feast day, September 26, is celebrated by hospitals and healthcare institutions, and their image is often displayed in hospitals and clinics.

Symbolism and Iconography

Cosmas and Damian are often depicted in art and iconography with a medicine chest and a staff, symbolizing their role as physicians and healers. They are also depicted with a red cross on their chest, symbolizing their martyrdom and their devotion to Christ.

Devotional Practices

Cosmas and Damian are honored through devotional practices such as prayer, meditation, and the recitation of the Rosary. Their intercession is sought by healthcare professionals, as well as by those who are sick or suffering. Many hospitals and healthcare institutions are named after them, and their image is often displayed in hospitals and clinics.

Miracles and Healings

Cosmas and Damian's intercession has been credited with numerous miracles and healings throughout history. Many people have reported experiencing their guidance and protection in their work, as well as their intercession in times of illness and suffering.

It is reassuring though, those almost two millennia after St. Cosmas and Damian, physicians and pharmacists continue to work together. A lesson we could learn from the brothers is that we should continue to support each other in our careers and together develop healthcare services for the benefit of our patients.

St. Cosmas and Damian are powerful patron saints for medicine, whose intercession and guidance are sought by many. Their selfless service and compassion towards the suffering have made them beloved figures in the history of the Church. Through their life and legacy, Cosmas and Damian remind us of the importance of charity, humility, and simplicity in serving the sick and the poor. Their feast day is a celebration of God's mercy and love for humanity, and their intercession is a source of comfort and strength for those who seek their aid.

Saint Pantaleon

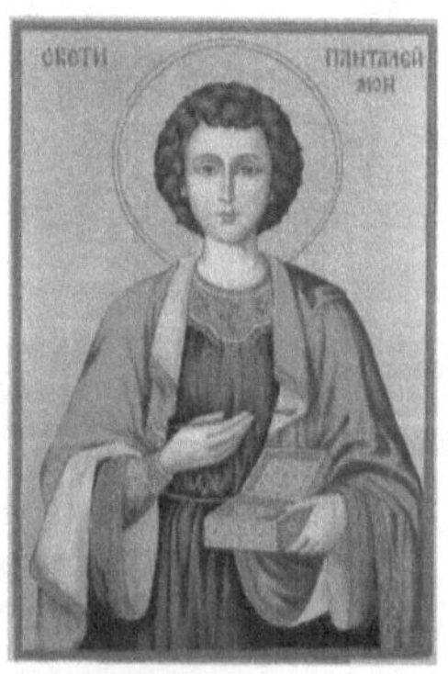

St. Pantaleon is a revered saint in the Catholic Church, known for his unwavering dedication to the sick and the poor. As a physician and martyr, he is revered as the patron saint of physicians, and his feast day, July 27, is celebrated by healthcare professionals around the world. His selfless service and compassion towards the suffering have made him a beloved figure in the history of the Church.

Early Life and Martyrdom

Saint Pantaleon (also known as Saint Panteleimon) is a revered figure in Christian tradition, known for his miraculous healing powers and his unwavering faith in the face of persecution. He is venerated as a patron saint of physicians, doctors, and midwives, and is considered a powerful intercessor for those in need of healing.

Pantaleon was born in Nicomedia, in modern-day Turkey, around 275 AD. He was raised in a wealthy pagan family and trained as a physician, mastering the art of medicine and surgery. Despite his success as a physician, Pantaleon was drawn to Christianity and became a devout follower of Christ.

As a Christian, Pantaleon used his medical knowledge to heal the sick, earning a reputation as a skilled physician and a compassionate caregiver. He also used his wealth to support the poor and needy, giving generously to those in need. Pantaleon's faith and his humanitarian work drew the ire of the Roman authorities, who were suspicious of Christians and their beliefs. When Emperor Diocletian began his persecution of Christians in 303 AD, Pantaleon was arrested and brought before the emperor.

Despite threats of torture and death, Pantaleon refused to renounce his faith, and instead proclaimed his belief in Christ and remained firm in his faith. He was subjected to brutal torture and ultimately martyred for his beliefs, dying a hero's death as a faithful witness to the Gospel.

In an art, Saint Pantaleon is depicted holding a cross, a book, and a medical instrument. He is also sometimes shown surrounded by children or animals. There are many churches dedicated to Saint Pantaleon throughout the world, including the Basilica of Saint Pantaleon in Cologne, Germany.

Patronage of Physicians

Pantaleon's dedication to the sick and the poor, as well as his martyrdom, have made him the patron saint of physicians. He is revered by healthcare professionals around the world, who seek his intercession and guidance in their work. His feast day is celebrated by hospitals and healthcare institutions, and his image is often displayed in hospitals and clinics.

Symbolism and Iconography

Pantaleon is often depicted in art and iconography with a medicine chest and a staff, symbolizing his role as a physician and healer. He is also depicted with a red cross on his chest, symbolizing his martyrdom and his devotion to Christ.

Miracles and Healings

Pantaleon's intercession has been credited with numerous miracles and healings throughout history. Many people have reported experiencing his guidance and protection in their work, as well as his intercession in times of illness and suffering.

In addition to his role as a patron saint of healing, Pantaleon is also associated with several miraculous events. According to legend, he was able to bring a dead child back to life, and he was also said to have miraculously healed a man with a broken leg. These stories have made Pantaleon a popular figure in Christian art and literature, and have inspired many to seek his intercession for healing and protection.

St. Pantaleon is a powerful patron saint for physicians, whose intercession and guidance are sought by many. His selfless service and compassion towards the suffering have made him a beloved figure in the history of the Church. Through his life and legacy, Pantaleon reminds us of the importance of charity, humility, and simplicity in serving the sick and the poor. His feast day is a celebration of God's mercy and love for humanity, and his intercession is a source of comfort and strength for those who seek his aid.

In addition to his patronage of physicians, Pantaleon is also revered as a protector against illness and disease. His intercession is sought by those who are suffering from physical or mental ailments, and his image is often displayed in homes and hospitals as a symbol of hope and healing. Pantaleon's legacy extends beyond his patronage of physicians and his intercession for the sick. He is also a model for all Christians, who are called to serve the Lord and their neighbors with compassion and love.

In conclusion, St. Pantaleon is a powerful patron saint for physicians, whose intercession and guidance are sought by many. His selfless service and compassion towards the suffering have made him a beloved figure in the history of the Church, and his legacy continues to inspire and uplift us today.

8. The Ethics of Medical Procedures

A Faith Based Perspective

This introduction sets the stage for exploring the complex intersections of Christian faith and medical procedures, and how Christians navigate these challenging issues with compassion, integrity, and faithfulness.

Christianity and medicine have a long and complex history, with many Christians playing a vital role in the development of healthcare and medical ethics. However, there are times when Christian beliefs and values come into conflict with certain medical procedures or treatments. This can lead to difficult decisions and ethical dilemmas for Christian patients, families, and healthcare providers.

Some examples of medical procedures that may conflict with Christian beliefs include:

- → Abortion and reproductive rights.

- → Euthanasia and end-of-life care.

- → Stem cell research and genetic engineering.

- → Gender reassignment surgery and transgender issues.

- → Blood transfusions and organ donation.

- → Contraception and family planning.

In these situations, Christians may turn to scripture, tradition, and church teaching for guidance. They may also seek counsel from clergy, ethicists, and healthcare professionals who share their faith and values.

Blood Transfusions

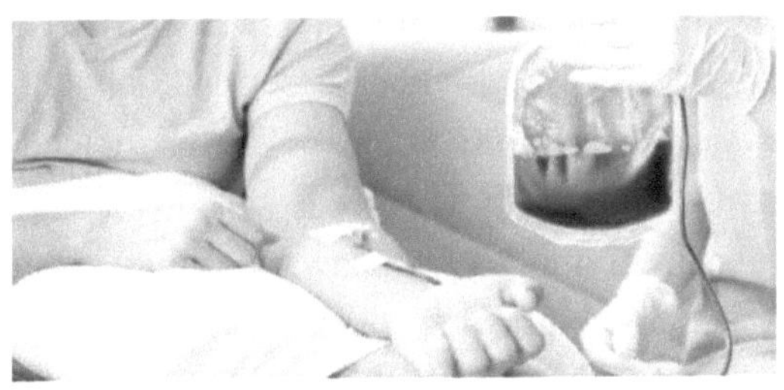

"Tears of a mother cannot save a child, but your blood can…"

The Catholic Church has a complex and evolving stance on blood transfusions, with a history spanning centuries. Initially, the Church opposed blood transfusions, citing concerns about the sanctity of human life and the potential for spiritual contamination. However, as medical understanding and technology advanced, the Church adapted its teachings to accommodate the life-saving benefits of blood transfusions.

In the 17th century, the first blood transfusions were performed, sparking debate among religious leaders. The Church initially prohibited blood transfusions, citing the biblical injunction against consuming blood (Genesis 9:4, Leviticus 17:10-14). This stance was reinforced by the 1679 decree *De Vita et Morte* by Pope Innocent XI, which condemned blood transfusions as "a type of cannibalism."

However, as the medical community continued to develop and refine blood transfusion techniques, the Church began to reconsider its stance. In the early 20th century, in 1948, Pope

Pius XII addressed a group of blood donors and compared their generosity in giving their blood with that of Jesus. He also addressed the same issue in his 1952 allocution *Optatam Totius*, stating that blood transfusions were morally acceptable when necessary to preserve human life. Similarly, in 1991, Pope John Paul II stated that, 'with blood transfusions, man has found a way to give of himself, of his blood... so that others may continue to live.' Pope Francis described the act of blood transfusion as, 'a testimony of love for our neighbor'. While Popes have repeatedly issued statements encouraging transfusion, many Catholics are unaware of these. Catholics may also be misled by contrasting claims found on the internet or even in books or journals.

The Church's shift in stance was further solidified by the 1980 statement from the Pontifical Academy of Sciences, which declared that "blood transfusions are in no way a violation of the biblical prohibition of ingesting blood." This statement acknowledged the distinction between consuming blood as food and receiving it as a life-saving medical treatment.

Today, the Catholic Church fully accepts blood transfusions as a legitimate and morally justifiable medical practice. The Church teaches that the decision to receive a blood transfusion should be made in consultation with medical professionals and in accordance with one's personal conscience.

In addition to its evolving stance on blood transfusions, the Catholic Church has also played a significant role in promoting blood donation and supporting blood banks. Many Catholic hospitals and organizations actively encourage blood donation, recognizing the critical importance of this life-saving resource.

In conclusion, the Catholic Church's stance on blood transfusions has undergone significant evolution over the centuries, from initial opposition to full acceptance. This shift reflects the Church's commitment in preserving human life and adapting to advances in medical technology and understanding. As the Church continues to engage with the medical community, its teachings on blood transfusions will likely continue to evolve, remaining grounded in the principles of respect for human life and the pursuit of compassionate care.

Euthanasia and Suicide

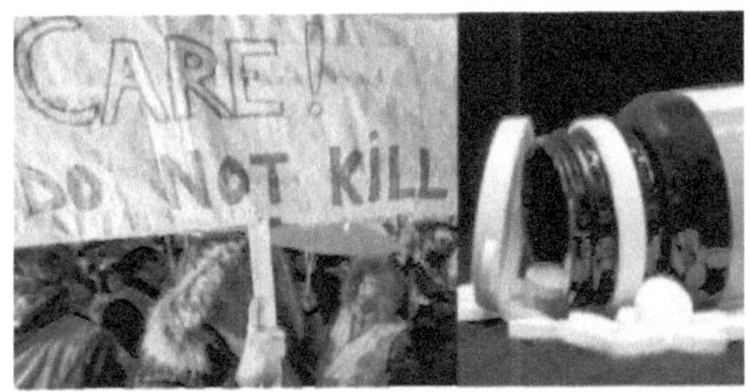

"Faith in resurrection helps us face death without fear"

The Catholic Church has a clear and unwavering stance on euthanasia and suicide, considering them grave moral evils that contradict the dignity and value of human life. This position is rooted in the Church's teaching on the sanctity of human life, which holds that every human being has inherent dignity and worth from conception to natural death.

The Church's opposition to euthanasia and suicide is based on its understanding of the Fifth Commandment, *Thou shalt not kill* (Exodus 20:13), and the teachings of the early Church Fathers, who consistently condemned suicide and euthanasia as a form of murder.

The Church's stance was formally articulated in Papal comments. In the encyclical *Mater et Magistra*, Pope John XXIII emphasized, "Human life is sacred. From its very inception it reveals the creating hand of God." And in the encyclical Pacem in terris, the same Pope, speaks of human rights, mentioned the right of all human beings to live, a right that "involves the duty to preserve one's life." The encyclical *Evangelium Vitae* by Pope John Paul II in 1995, emphasized the Church's opposition to euthanasia, suicide, and assisted suicide as-"Here we are faced with one of the more alarming symptoms of the 'culture of death'."

Pope Francis underlined the point in 2017, in a Message to members of the World Medical Association: "It is clear that not adopting, or else suspending, disproportionate measures, means avoiding overzealous treatment; from an ethical standpoint, it is completely different from euthanasia, which is always wrong, in that the intent of euthanasia is to end life and cause death." And he recalled the teaching of the Catechism of the Catholic Church (2278), "Discontinuing medical procedures that are burdensome, dangerous, extraordinary, or disproportionate to the expected outcome can be legitimate; it is the refusal of 'over-zealous' treatment. Here one does not will to cause death; one's inability to impede it is merely accepted."

In the Letter *Samaritanus bonus*, approved by Pope Francis and published in September 2020, the Congregation for the Doctrine of the Faith affirms, "The judgement that an illness is incurable cannot mean that care has come at an end." Those who are suffering from a terminal illness, as well as babies born with a limited expectation of survival have the right to be welcomed, cared for, and surrounded by affection. The Church "reaffirms as definitive teaching that euthanasia is a crime against human life."

In keeping with the Catholic Church's vision, suicide is an objectively sinful act. On this basis, euthanasia is gravely sinful for both the person who will die and the person who assists to bring about their death. Instead of deliberately killing our aged and dying, we should work together to secure the common good.

The Catholic Church teaches that human life is a gift from God and should be cherished and protected, even in the face of suffering and illness. The Church encourages patients, families, and healthcare providers to pursue palliative care and hospice services that prioritize comfort, dignity, and compassion, rather than resorting to euthanasia or assisted suicide.

In addition to its moral opposition to euthanasia and suicide, the Catholic Church has also played a significant role in providing healthcare and end-of-life care services that prioritize the dignity and worth of every human person. The Church's healthcare ministries often emphasize the importance of compassionate care, spiritual support, and accompaniment for patients and families facing serious illness and death.

Some critics argue that the Church's stance on euthanasia and suicide is overly rigid and neglects the complexities of real-life situations, such as cases of unbearable suffering or terminal illness. However, the Church maintains that its teaching on the sanctity of human life is rooted in its understanding of the inherent dignity and worth of every human person, regardless of circumstances.

The Church also recognizes the importance of addressing issues related to mental health, depression, and suicide prevention, particularly among young people and vulnerable populations. The Church's mental health ministries often prioritize early intervention, support services, and community resources to help individuals struggling with mental health issues.

In conclusion, the Catholic Church's stance on euthanasia and suicide is clear and unwavering, recognizing the inherent dignity and worth of every human person and encouraging compassionate care, spiritual support, and accompaniment for patients and families facing serious illness and death. While the Church's position may be seen as controversial or rigid by some, it remains a core aspect of Catholic teaching and a guiding principle for the Church's healthcare and end-of-life care services.

Contraception and Family Planning

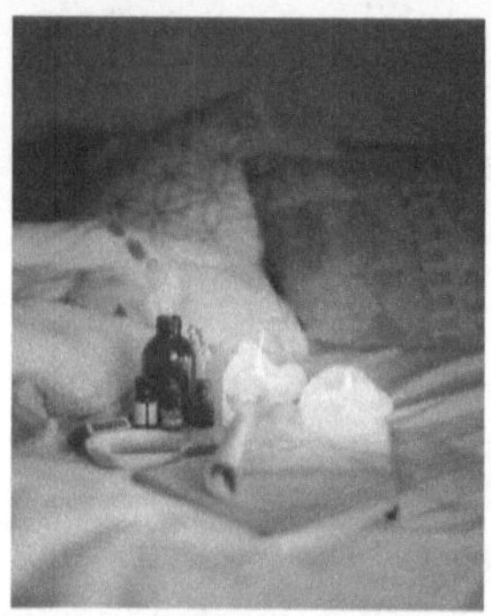

"Be fruitful and multiply and fill the Earth" –
Genesis 9:11

The Catholic Church has a complex and nuanced stance on family planning and contraception, with a history spanning centuries. While the Church teaches that married couples should be open to life and cherish children, it also recognizes the importance of responsible parenthood and the need for couples to make informed decisions about their family size.

Historically, the Church has prohibited artificial contraception, citing its opposition to the separation of the unitive and procreative aspects of sexual intercourse. This stance was formally articulated in the 1968 encyclical *Humanae Vitae* by Pope Paul VI, which reaffirmed the Church's teaching against artificial contraception.

However, the Church also acknowledges the importance of Natural Family Planning (NFP) methods, which involve tracking a woman's fertility cycles to avoid or achieve pregnancy. NFP methods are seen as a morally acceptable way for couples to regulate their fertility, as they do not involve the use of artificial contraceptives.

The Bible also specifically extols the value of children. "Behold, children are a heritage from the Lord, the fruit of the womb a reward" (Psalm 127:3). Children should be highly valued, and should be seen as gifts to us. Seeing children as just the by-products of sex is very detrimental and violates the spirit of such biblical texts. With all this in mind, it is also crucial to see that truly caring for a child means making wise decisions so that one has the means, including emotional investment, financial resources, and time, to give good care. This may mean that a couple limits the number of children they have in order to best provide for each child's emotional, physical, and spiritual needs.

Of course, God is the ultimate Master; He can choose to bring a life into the world anytime He chooses, even if it defies human wisdom. It appears, however, that God has granted parents the responsibility for family planning. He has commanded His people, particularly in the books of Proverbs and Ecclesiastes, to make wise decisions, and this extends to building a family (Campbell, 1960). So we must decide what responsible family decision-making looks like.

Just as childbearing is not the only purpose for sex, having children is not the defining feature of a marriage. God commands his people to "Be fruitful and multiply" (Genesis 1:28), and procreation is an important part of humans' mandate. However, "the idea that Christian hope is in eternal life rather than in many generations of their own genetic offspring is crucial. A marriage without children is already a true marriage because of the God-given nature of the covenant relationship".

However, some couples may choose artificial methods of birth control, such as barrier or certain hormonal methods. Since these two methods are not abortive, they should not be ethically forbidden for all Christians. The Catholic Church only permits NFP because it does not completely block the procreative aspect of sex.

In recent years, the Church has emphasized the importance of responsible parenthood and the need for couples to make informed decisions about their family size. Pope Francis has spoken about the need for couples to be responsible and generous in their decisions about family size, while also acknowledging the importance of discernment and prayer in making these decisions.

Despite its opposition to artificial contraception, the Catholic Church has also recognized the importance of addressing issues related to population growth and sustainable development. The Church has called for increased access to education and healthcare, particularly for women and children, as a way to address these issues in a morally responsible and sustainable way.

Some critics argue that the Church's stance on contraception is outdated and neglects the realities of modern life, particularly in regards to issues such as overpopulation and poverty. However, the Church maintains that its teaching on contraception is rooted in its understanding of human sexuality and the importance of upholding the dignity and worth of every human person.

In addition to its moral opposition to artificial contraception, the Catholic Church has also played a significant role in providing healthcare and family planning services to communities around the world. The Church's healthcare ministries often prioritize natural family planning methods and provide education and support for couples making decisions about their family size.

In conclusion, the Catholic Church's stance on family planning and contraception is complex and nuanced, recognizing the importance of responsible parenthood and the need for couples to make informed decisions about their family size. While the Church maintains its opposition to artificial contraception, it also acknowledges the importance of addressing issues related to population growth and sustainable development, and provides healthcare and family planning services to communities around the world.

Organ Donation

"Be a symbol of hope for those who are waiting"

The Catholic Church has a positive stance on organ donation, considering it a selfless act of charity and a way to promote the common good. This position is rooted in the Church's teaching on the dignity of the human person and the importance of showing compassion and love for one's neighbor.

Pope John Paul II, in his Address to the 18th International Congress of the Transplantation Society (2000) said, "…There is a need to instill in people's hearts, especially in the hearts of the young, a genuine and deep appreciation of the need for brotherly love, a love that can find expression in the decision to become an organ donor."

In 2000, the Pontifical Academy of Sciences issued a statement supporting organ donation, stating that "the donation of organs after death is a noble and meritorious act that can be a sign of love and solidarity with others." The Church encourages Catholics to consider organ donation as a way to give the gift of life to others, even after their own passing.

Christians value the body as the temple of the Holy Spirit (1 Corinthians 6:19) and look forward to a resurrection of the body at the end of time. Yet, it is the Christian belief that nothing that happens to our body, before or after death, can impact our relationship with God: "For I know that my Redeemer lives… and after my skin has been thus destroyed, then from my flesh I shall see God, whom I shall see on my side, and my eyes shall behold," (Job 19:25-27) roman Catholics view organ and tissue donation as an act of charity and love.

The Ethical and Religious Directives for Catholic Health Care Services, a set of principles that guide the healing mission of the Church, clearly explains the permissibility of organ donations. In Directive No. 30, we read: "The transplantation of organs from living donors is morally permissible when such a donation will not sacrifice or seriously impair any essential bodily function and the anticipated benefit to the recipient is proportionate to the harm to the donor." Similarly, Directives No. 63-66 treat organ donation as follows: Directive No. 63: "Catholic health care institutions should encourage and provide the means whereby those who wish to do so may arrange for the donation of their organs and bodily tissue, for ethically legitimate purposes, so that they may be used for donation and research after death." Directive No. 64: "Such organs should not be removed until it has been medically determined that the patient has died. In order to prevent any conflict of interest, the physician who determines death should not be a member of the transplant team."

. It is the Church's position that transplanted organs never be offered for sale. They are to be given as a gift of love. Any procedure that commercializes or considers organs as items for exchange or trade is morally unacceptable. The decision as to who should have priority in regards to organ transplantation must be based solely on medical factors and not on such considerations as age, sex, religion, social standing or other similar standards.

In addition, it is of the utmost importance that informed consent by the donor and/or donor's legitimate representatives be had and that vital organs, those that occur singly in the body, are removed only after certain death (the complete and irreversible cessation of all brain activity) has occurred.

The Church's support for organ donation is based on its understanding of the human body as a temple of the Holy Spirit (1 Corinthians 6:19-20) and the importance of treating it with respect and dignity, even after death. The Church also recognizes the importance of promoting the common good and supporting the well-being of others, particularly those in need of life-saving transplants.

Some critics have raised concerns about the Church's stance on organ donation, particularly regarding issues such as the definition of death and the potential for coercion or exploitation. However, the Church has addressed these concerns through its teachings and guidelines, emphasizing the importance of informed consent, respect for the donor's autonomy, and the need for ethical and responsible practices in organ donation.

In addition to its moral support for organ donation, the Catholic Church has also played a significant role in promoting organ donation awareness and education, particularly through its healthcare ministries and institutions. Many Catholic hospitals and healthcare organizations have implemented organ donation programs and protocols, prioritizing the importance of organ donation and supporting families and patients in their decisions.

The Church's encouragement of organ donation is also reflected in its teachings on the importance of caring for others and promoting the common good. Pope Francis has emphasized the need for solidarity and compassion in addressing the needs of others, particularly those who are vulnerable and marginalized. Organ donation is seen as a tangible expression of this solidarity and compassion, offering a chance to give life and hope to others.

In conclusion, the Catholic Church's stance on organ donation is one of support and encouragement, recognizing the importance of promoting the common good and showing compassion and love for one's neighbor. While the Church has addressed concerns and ethical considerations, its teaching on organ donation emphasizes the dignity and respect due to the human person, even after death, and the importance of promoting life and hope for others.

In Vitro Fertilization

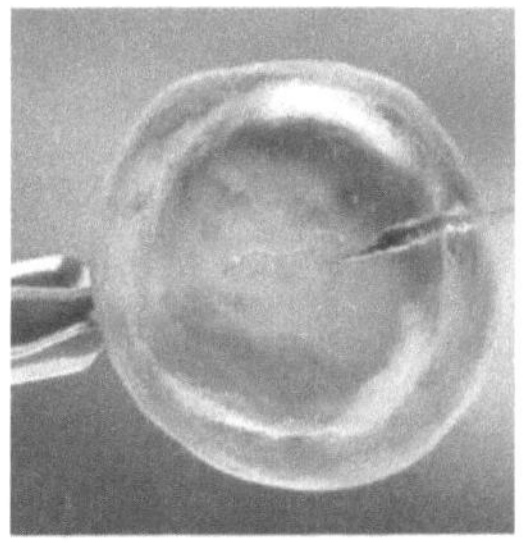

"God values every life; he creates and plans for every birth"

In vitro fertilization is a method by which a male's sperm and a female's eggs are collected by a physician then mixed in a petri dish in the hopes that one or more of the eggs will become fertilized. Science teaches us that, from the very first moment an egg is fertilized, it becomes an embryo — and an unrepeatable human being now exists.

The Catholic Church has consistently taken a stance against In Vitro Fertilization (IVF), viewing it as a morally objectionable practice that goes against the natural law and the teachings of the Church. According to the Church, human life is sacred and should be respected from the moment of conception to natural death. The use of IVF, which involves the creation of human embryos outside the human body, is seen as a violation of this principle.

Genesis 1:28 says: "God blessed them and God said to them: Be fertile and multiply; fill the earth and subdue it." The Catechism of the Catholic Church teaches us that "by its very nature the institution of marriage and married love is ordered to the procreation and education of the offspring and it is in them that it finds its crowning glory. Children are the supreme gift of marriage and contribute greatly to the good of the parents themselves." It is therefore only natural that couples long to have children.

For many, the desire to have a child, or many children, is immense. Children are wonderful blessings. Children give us hope for the future. Children make families whole. And, for most people, this desire for children is easily fulfilled. But what happens when that desire to have a child results in negative pregnancy test after negative pregnancy test? That void in a mother's or father's life—and in their hearts—seems bottomless. They begin to feel despair, a lack of hope, and desperation.

It is this despair, coupled with the fierce desire to conceive, that leads people to seek out the help of in vitro fertilization to create a child. After all, they think, why does it matter how our child is created if we love and take care of him? However, the catechism and our faith teach us that it does matter.

The Church teaches that the only moral way to conceive a child is through the loving embrace of the marital act. The dignity of the child requires this of us. This beautiful, wonderful expression of love between the husband and the wife works in cooperation with God to create a totally separate human being. That is why we call it procreation rather than creation.

According to *Donum Vitae*, IVF is considered sinful partly because it dissociates the sexual act from the procreative act. The act that brings the child into existence is no longer an act by which two persons give themselves fully to one another under God's embrace, but instead it "entrusts the life and identity of the embryo into the power of doctors and biologists and establishes the domination of technology over the origin and destiny of the human person.Such a relationship of domination is in itself contrary to the dignity and equality that must be common to parents and children."

As the Catechism of the Catholic Church teaches, Techniques that entail the dissociation of husband and wife, by the intrusion of a person other than the couple (e.g., donation of sperm or ovum, surrogate uterus), are gravely immoral. These techniques (heterologous artificial insemination and fertilization) infringe on the child's right to be born of a father and mother known to him and bound to each other by marriage. They betray the spouses' "right to become a father and a mother only through each other."

We must also understand that every child possesses genuine rights: the right "to be the fruit of the specific act of the conjugal love of his parents," and "the right to be respected as a person from the moment of his conception."

In 2008, the Congregation for the Doctrine of the Faith wrote about the dignity of the person in *Dignitas Personae*. It stated: "The blithe acceptance of the enormous number of abortions involved in the process of in vitro fertilization vividly illustrates how the replacement of the conjugal act by a technical procedure – in addition to being in contradiction with the respect that is due to procreation as something that cannot be reduced to mere reproduction – leads to a weakening of the respect owed to every human being."

Children are not a given. They are "the supreme gift of marriage" (CCC 2378). When children are created within the confines of a petri dish, they become a commodity.

As human beings created in the image and likeness of God, we are never to be something bought or sold. God freely gives us life, and we are to cherish that life, never profit from it or purchase it. We must never put a price on a human being, but that is exactly what IVF does. At around $15,000 to $20,000 per round of IVF, this medical procedure often sucks bank accounts dry, depletes retirement accounts, and takes advantage of desperate potential parents. And, with a success rate at only about 42% for women under 35—and much less for older women—IVF is no guarantee or easy solution.

Setting cost aside, let's look at what happens when embryos are created in a dish. A doctor will determine which of these embryos have the greatest potential to grow further if implanted, so he will choose those. That leaves the remaining ones to be either frozen or discarded. After a few potential embryos have been selected, the parents can choose how many will be implanted in the mother's uterus.

If, for example, five babies were deemed to have the best potential, the mother might choose to have three implanted and save the other two for a future time. If the parents so desire, these remaining embryos will then be frozen. But they have other options as well, including donating them to another infertile couple (CCC 2376), donating them to science for research, and disposing of them.

All of these instances are highly immoral. For instance, any of those "extras" – having been fertilized – are human beings. Generally, multiple embryos are implanted because not all of them (or any) may "take." Sometimes, if multiple babies have attached and begun to grow, the doctor may even suggest that "extras" be eliminated for the good growth of one or two. Any "disposal" of embryos is an early abortion.

None of these options afford a baby the dignity and respect he deserves as a child of God. Furthermore, when we use science to create children, we are usurping the role of God and putting our wants and desires above His. We are telling Him that we do not trust His plans and those we refuse to follow His laws in search of our own selfish desires.

Babies created in IVF labs are human beings. They are somebody's children. They have souls. To discard them, give them up for research, or to leave them frozen indefinitely is a sickening prospect.

The Church understands the anxiety and the grief that come with infertility. And Catholic ministries like Springs in the Desert and The Fruitful Hollow are available to offer solace and peace during these difficult times. These groups provide resources, small group meetings, and information about moral treatments for couples facing infertility.

One such place that offers ethical treatment for infertile couples is the Pope Paul VI Institute for the Study of Human Reproduction. According to its website, its natural techniques "provide effective, morally acceptable, and sexually healthy options for women and couples" so that they can achieve a successful pregnancy.

The mission of the Institute is to help couples achieve fertility through morally licit means. These treatments include ovulation drugs, surgeries, and a technique called NaProTECHNOLOGY (natural procreative technology)—a technology that helps women monitor and maintain their reproductive health—to remedy problems created by conditions such as endometriosis, pelvic adhesions, polycystic ovarian disease, obstructions of the fallopian tubes, hormonal dysfunctions, and more. The institute explains that many of these underlying conditions can be treated so that the couple can conceive a child naturally rather than having to resort to IVF. The Saint Paul VI's Institute's tremendous success with patients is even greater than the success rate of IVF.

The devastation, the loneliness, and the sadness that couples feel when they cannot conceive a child is real, and we should pray daily for them and encourage them to pray for the intercession of saints such as St. Gerard, St. Rita, and St. Gianna Molla. But we must remember that the desire to have a child cannot take precedence over the life of a human being. Our faith calls us to cherish and respect life—at all stages—even in its tiniest form.

Abortion

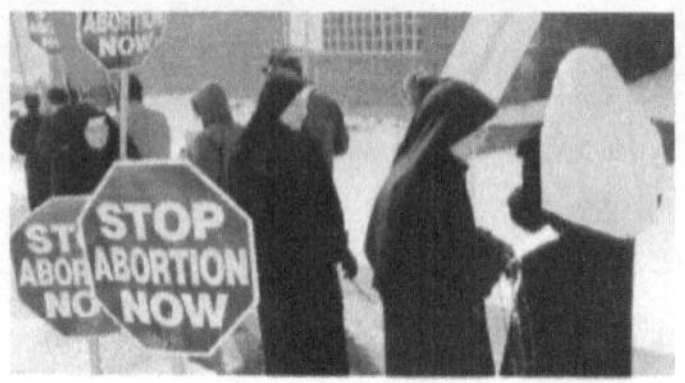

"See each child as a gift to be welcomed, cherished and protected"

The Catholic Church has a longstanding and unwavering stance on abortion, condemning it as a grave moral evil. This position is rooted in the Church's teaching on the sanctity of human life, which holds that every human being has inherent dignity and worth from conception to natural death.

The Church's opposition to abortion is based on its understanding of the Fifth Commandment, "Thou shalt not kill" (Exodus 20:13), and the teachings of the early Church Fathers, who consistently condemned abortion as a form of infanticide. The Church's stance was formally articulated in the 14th century by St. Thomas Aquinas, who argued that abortion is a violation of the natural law and the divine plan for human life.

In modern times, the Church's teaching on abortion has been reaffirmed and developed through various papal encyclicals and statements from the Magisterium. The 1968 encyclical *"Humanae Vitae"* by Pope Paul VI emphasized the Church's opposition to abortion, as well as artificial contraception and sterilization. The 1995 encyclical *Evangelium Vitae* by Pope John Paul II further clarified the Church's stance, stating that "direct abortion, that is, abortion willed as an end or as a means to an end, is gravely contrary to the moral law" (EV 62).

The Catholic Church's teaching on abortion is grounded in its understanding of the human person as a unique and precious creation of God, imbued with inherent dignity and worth. The Church believes that every human life has value and should be protected and cherished, from the moment of conception to natural death.

In addition to its moral opposition to abortion, the Catholic Church has also played a significant role in supporting pregnant women and families through various ministries and organizations. The Church's pro-life efforts aim to provide alternatives to abortion, such as adoption and support services for pregnant women, as well as advocacy for policies that protect human life and dignity.

Some critics argue that the Church's stance on abortion is overly rigid and neglects the complexities of real-life situations, such as cases of rape or incest. However, the Church's teaching emphasizes the inherent value and dignity of every human life, regardless of circumstances. The Church also recognizes the importance of compassion and support for women facing difficult pregnancies, while maintaining its moral opposition to abortion.

9. Prayerful Moments

Collection of Medical Prayers

Prayer has long been a cornerstone of human experience, providing comfort, solace, and strength in times of need. In the context of healthcare, prayer plays a vital role in the well-being and recovery of patients, families, and healthcare providers alike. From the bedside to the operating room, prayer can be a powerful tool in the healing process. Healthcare providers, patients, and families can all benefit from the comfort and strength that prayer provides. This exploration of the role of prayer in healthcare invites us to examine the ways in which faith and medicine intersect, and how prayer can be a vital part of the healing journey.

Healthcare professionals, including doctors, nurses, and other medical staff, often play a critical role in the physical and emotional well-being of their patients. In addition to providing medical care, many healthcare professionals also recognize the importance of spiritual care and the power of prayer in the healing process. By incorporating prayer into their practice, healthcare professionals can demonstrate their commitment to comprehensive care, recognizing the intricate relationship between body, mind, and spirit.

Prayer for Healing By Patients

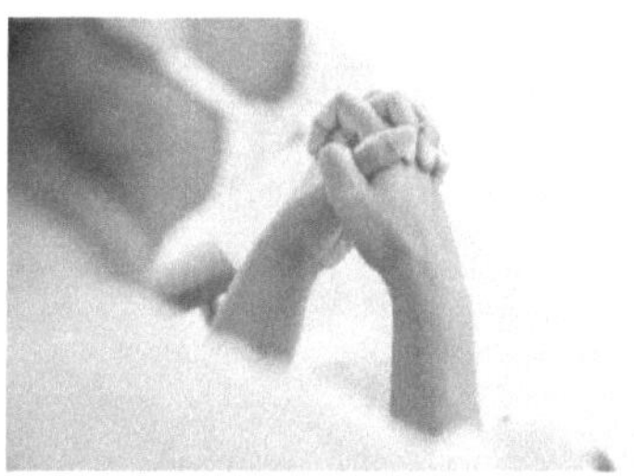

This prayer reflects Christian beliefs and values, such as:

✓ Trusting in God's love and care.

✓ Seeking refuge and strength in God.

✓ Asking for healing and comfort.

✓ Trusting in God's sovereignty.

✓ Seeking forgiveness and surrendering worries and doubts.

✓ Glorifying God in suffering.

✓ Trusting in God's goodness and promises.

"Dear God,

I come to you in need, trusting in your love and care. Please be my refuge and strength in this time of illness or uncertainty. Lord Jesus, you healed the sick and comforted the afflicted. I ask for your healing touch, your comfort, and your peace. Holy Spirit, guides my medical team with wisdom and skill, and helps me to trust in your sovereignty. Forgive me for any sins or fears that may be hindering my healing. Help me to surrender my worries and doubts to you. I pray for your will to be done in my life, even in the midst of this challenge. May I glorify you in my suffering and trust in your goodness. Thank you for your promise to be with me always, and for the hope of eternal life through Jesus Christ. In his name, I pray. Amen."

Prayer for Service by Medical Professionals

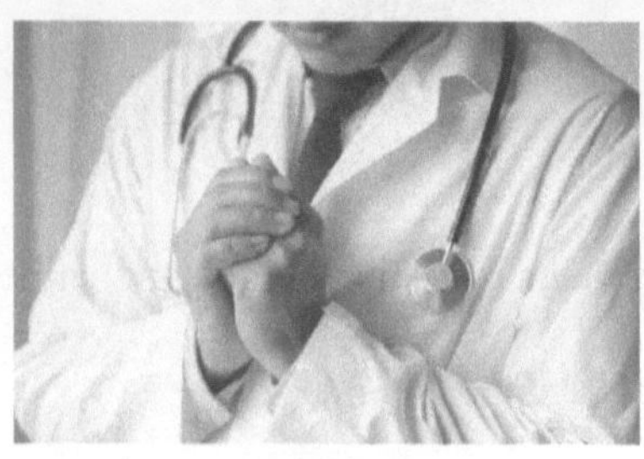

Tips to Offer Prayer

1. Start with gratitude: Express thanks for the privilege of serving others through medicine.

2. Ask for guidance: Seek wisdom and discernment in diagnosis, treatment, and patient care.

3. Pray for patients: Lift up patients by name, asking for healing, comfort, and peace.

4. Request strength and compassion: Ask God to renew your energy and empathy, especially in challenging situations.

5. Seek spiritual guidance: Pray for wisdom in navigating ethical dilemmas and difficult decisions.

6. Offer your work to God: Dedicate your skills and expertise to His service, asking that your work honor Him.

7. Pray for colleagues and staff: Ask God to bless and guide your team, promoting unity and harmony.

8. Find peace in God's sovereignty: Trust that God is in control, even in uncertain or difficult situations.

9. Pray for personal growth: Ask God to shape you into a better servant, friend, and follower of Jesus.

10. End with praise: Affirm God's goodness, love, and faithfulness, regardless of circumstances.

"Dear God, thank you for the privilege of serving others through medicine. Guide me in my work today, granting wisdom and compassion. I lift up my patients to you, asking for healing and peace. Renew my strength and energy, and help me navigate challenging situations with grace and wisdom. May my work honor you, and may I always find peace in your sovereignty. Amen."

Prayer for Knowledge by Medical Students

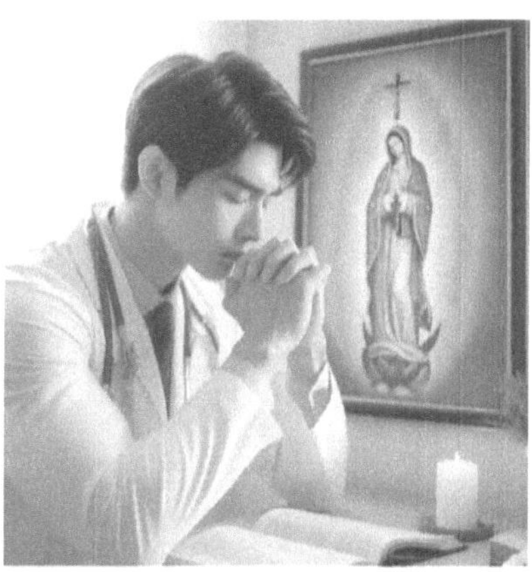

This prayer reflects Christian beliefs and values, such as:

- Gratitude for the opportunity to serve others.

- Seeking guidance and wisdom from God.

- Following Jesus' example of compassion and love.

- Trusting in the Holy Spirit for knowledge and discernment.

- Glorifying God in all aspects of life and work.

"Dear Heavenly Father,

We come before you today as medical students, grateful for the opportunity to serve others in your name. We ask for your guidance and wisdom as we study and prepare to care for your children. Lord Jesus, you healed the sick, comforted the afflicted, and loved the unlovable. Help us to follow your example, to see each patient as a beloved child of God, and to treat them with compassion, kindness, and respect. Holy Spirit, grant us knowledge, skill, and discernment as we navigate the complexities of medicine. Help us to stay grounded in your truth, to seek your wisdom, and to trust in your sovereignty. May our studies be fruitful, our patients be healed, and our hearts be filled with love and joy. May we always remember that our gifts and talents come from you, and that our ultimate goal is to glorify you in all we do. We pray this in the name of Jesus Christ, our Lord and Xavior. Amen."

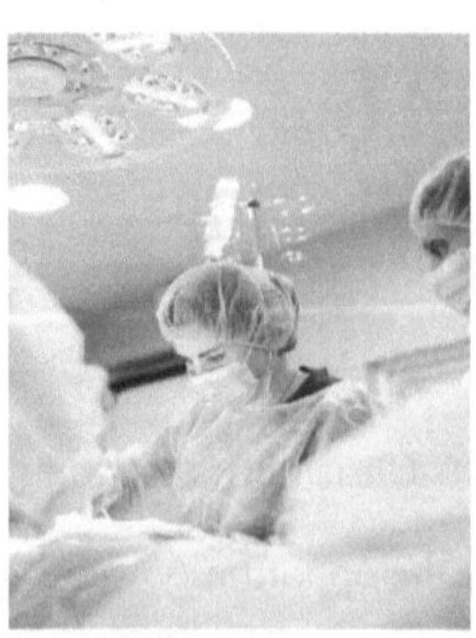

Bibliography

1. Ellen G White 2021, The Ministry of Healing Paperback by Notion Press.

2. Paul Zinter 2007 A Time to Heal The Biblical Ministry of Divine Healing by Xulon Press.

3. Mother Teresa 2002 Book Of Peace, The Paperback by Rider press.

4. Mother Teresa: Come Be My Light Paperback – 7 August 2008 by Brian Kolodiejchuk Rider & Co.

5. Florence Nightingale: The Courageous Life of the Legendary Nurse Hardcover – Import, 21 November 2016 by Catherine Reef Mariner Books, US.

6. Florence Nightingale: A Life Inspired Paperback – Import, 17 April 2015 by Lynn M. Hamilton (Author), Wyatt North Createspace Independent Pub.

7. Clara Barton: Courage to Serve (Heroes of History) Hardcover – Illustrated, 1 December 2007 by Renee Taft Meloche (Author), Bryan Pollard, Emerald Books, U.S.

8. Ida Scudder: Missionary Doctor Kindle Edition by Terri B. Kelly BJU Press/JourneyForth (8 August 2021).

9. Ida Scudder: Healing Bodies, Touching Hearts (Christian Heroes: Then & Now) Kindle Edition by Janet Benge (Author), Geoff Benge YWAM Publishing (31 May 2012).

10. The Christian Virtues in Medical Practice By Edmund D. Pellegrino MD, David C. Thomasma • 1996 Georgetown University Press.

11. The Diseases of the Bible By Risdon Bennett • 2023 Creative Media Partners, LLC.

12. The Diseases of the Bible By Andrew Dickson White, James Risdon Bennett • 2015 Creative Media Partners, LLC.

13. The Bible and Medicinal Plants The Healing Power of Natural Medicines By Mohamad Hesam Shahrajabian, Ted Trandahl • 2021 Nova Medicine & Health.

14. Healing Plants of the Bible History, Lore & Meditations By Vincenzina Krymow • 2002 Wild Goose.

15. Voice of a Stranger ... Missionary Endeavour in India By Ruth Dibble • 1975 Ludhiana Brit. Fellowship.

16. Men of Might in India Missions The Leaders and Their Epochs, 1706-1899 By Helen Harriet Holcomb • 1901 Young People's Missionary Movement.

17. Ida S. Scudder of Vellore The Life Story of Ida Sophia Scudder By Mary Pauline Jeffery • 1951 Wesley Press.

18. The Medical Mission Its Place, Power and Appeal By Sir William James Wanless • 1911 Westminster Press.

19. Dear and Glorious Physician A Novel About Saint Luke By Taylor Caldwell • 2024 Open Road Media.

20. Raphael Communicating with the Archangel for Healing & Creativity By Richard Webster • 2012 Llewellyn Worldwide, Limited.

21. Camillus De Lellis The Hospital Saint By Mary Camilla Lyons • 2023 Creative Media Partners, LLC Medical Saints.

22. Cosmas and Damian in a Postmodern World By Jacalyn Duffin • 2013 OUP USA.

23. Blood Transfusions A History and Evaluation of the Religions, Biblical and Medical Objections By Jerry Bergman • 1994 Witness, Incorporated.

24. Dying to Kill A Christian Perspective on Euthanasia and Assisted Suicide By Kieran Beville • 2014 Christian Publishing House.

25. Contraception A History of Its Treatment by the Catholic Theologians and Canonists, Enlarged Edition By John T. Noonan, Jr., John Thomas Noonan • 2012 Harvard University Press.

26. Harvesting Organs & Cherishing Life What Christians Need to Know About Organ Donation and Procurement By Bogosh C Klessig H • 2021 Amazon Digital Services LLC – Kdp.

27. Abortion A Christian Understanding and Response James Karl Hoffmeier 1987 Baker Book House.

28. Whispers of Healing Prayers for Doctors: Doctors Prayer Book: Prayers for Medical Professionals - Thoughtful Appreciation Gift For Doctors - Give Your Christian Doctor The Gift Of Strength In Faith By Prayer Power Publishing • 2023 Amazon Digital Services LLC – Kdp.

29. Conceived by Science Thinking Carefully and Compassionately about Infertility and IVF 2021 By Stephanie Gray Connors.

Citations

1. Healthcare professionals have the great privilege and responsibility of serving the sick, and this allows us to revive and enrich our calling in unity with our Lord.

    – Dr Marta Kokoszynska.

2. Let us understand that God is a physician and each suffering is a medicine for salvation, not a punishment for damnation.

    – St Augustine.

3. The good physician treats the disease; the great physician treats the patient who has the disease.

    – William Oster.

4. Wherever the art of medicine is loved, there is also a love for humanity.

    – Hippocrates.

5. Take care of your health, that it may serve you to serve God.

    – St Francis De Sales.

6. Being healthcare providers means to hold all your tears and start drawing smiles on patients faces.

    – Dana Basem.

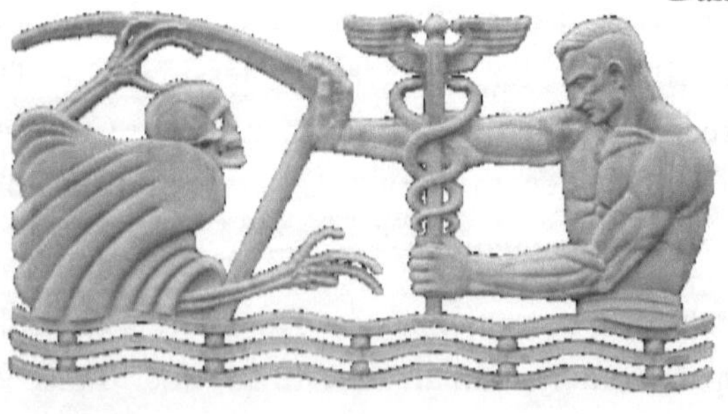